Updates in Surgery

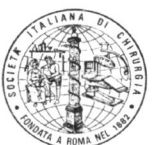

The aim of this series is to provide informative updates on hot topics in the areas of breast, endocrine, and abdominal surgery, surgical oncology, and coloproctology, and on new surgical techniques such as robotic surgery, laparoscopy, and minimally invasive surgery. Readers will find detailed guidance on patient selection, performance of surgical procedures, and avoidance of complications. In addition, a range of other important aspects are covered, from the role of new imaging tools to the use of combined treatments and postoperative care.

The topics addressed by volumes in the series Updates in Surgery have been selected for their broad significance in collaboration with the Italian Society of Surgery. Each volume will assist surgical residents and fellows and practicing surgeons in reaching appropriate treatment decisions and achieving optimal outcomes. The series will also be highly relevant for surgical researchers.

More information about this series at http://www.springer.com/series/8147

Marco Montorsi
Editor

Volume-Outcome Relationship in Oncological Surgery

In collaboration with Matteo Donadon

Forewords by
Paolo De Paolis
Pierpaolo Sileri

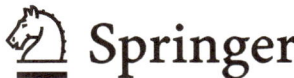 Springer

Editor
Marco Montorsi
Department of Biomedical Sciences
Humanitas University
Pieve Emanuele
Milan
Italy

Department of General Surgery
Humanitas Clinical and Research Center IRCCS
Rozzano
Milan
Italy

The publication and the distribution of this volume have been supported by the Italian Society of Surgery

ISSN 2280-9848   ISSN 2281-0854   (electronic)
Updates in Surgery
ISBN 978-3-030-51805-9   ISBN 978-3-030-51806-6   (eBook)
https://doi.org/10.1007/978-3-030-51806-6

Revision and editing: R. M. Martorelli, Scienzaperta (Novate Milanese, Italy)

This Springer imprint is published by the registered company Springer Nature Switzerland AG
The registered company address is: Gewerbestrasse 11, 6330 Cham, Switzerland

Foreword

Despite the body of literature in favor of the volume-outcome relationship and of the consequent centralization of high-risk operations, many aspects require further investigation. It is therefore a real pleasure for me to introduce this important book, for which Marco Montorsi engaged other world-renowned authors, whose experience and scientific excellence have produced a complete collection of contributions in this debated field.

Particular attention is paid to the core outcome set in surgical oncology, focusing on the selection of appropriate outcomes in clinical research and stressing not only their proper evaluation but also the need for the findings to be easily translated to practice and to be useful, reliable, and relevant to patients, healthcare professionals, and others involved in making decisions regarding healthcare provision.

This volume also highlights the strategic role of AGENAS in the development of oncological networks in Italy and the volume-outcome relationship in the different fields of surgery: esophageal, hepatobiliary, pancreatic, colorectal, soft tissue sarcomas, breast, endocrine, and robotic.

The importance of combining risk management and real-time indicator monitoring is also extensively discussed, as well as the mutual relationship between centralization and the accreditation process.

The volume is exhaustive in every aspect and it should represent a point of reference for every surgeon. On behalf of the Italian Society of Surgery, I would like to thank all the eminent authors who collaborated in producing this important monograph.

Turin, Italy
September 2020

Paolo De Paolis
Italian Society of Surgery
Turin, Italy

Foreword

This new volume addresses a unique topic on the balance between outcomes and volumes in oncological surgery. Is 'The more I do, the better I do' really true? For everyone, anywhere, and for any patient who experiences a diagnosis of cancer? The editor has had the intuition to address a challenging topic, delivering responses to the needs of all involved in the fight against cancer. The editor has put together a team of authors from among leading clinicians as well as institutions and patients' representatives to provide a critical and exhaustive overview of this issue.

Readers will immediately gain a clear image and definite answers to some open questions on the correlation between volumes and outcomes. Pros and cons, current practices, results, scientific evidence, and necessary strategies are all discussed with extraordinary harmony.

High standards and excellent results are obtained only by creating networks and investing in an adequately trained and skilled workforce. Clinical networks are mandatory not only as a monitoring tool, but also to enhance training, facilitate research, and lead political and regulatory activities ranging from prevention to management. All these actions guarantee year after year superior oncological results while we are all engaged in contrasting the dramatic rise of the global cancer burden.

This inspiring volume represents a useful tool that should be present on our desk to guide us in our daily practice.

Rome, Italy
September 2020

Pierpaolo Sileri
Deputy Minister of Health
Rome, Italy

Preface

The series *Updates in Surgery,* published by Springer, represents one of the master-pieces of the editorial activities of the Italian Society of Surgery; the aim has always been to present both its members and the national and international surgical community with monographic volumes which take stock of current and at times somewhat controversial issues.

Therefore, I would like to thank the Board of Directors of the Society not only for identifying and investigating this important area for the first time but also for entrusting the task to me as editor.

The relationship between the volume of surgical activity and clinical outcome is not a new topic and it was first dealt with in the surgical literature in the late 1970s. Subsequent contributions, particularly from the USA and later from other European settings, enabled the accrual of data demonstrating a positive correlation between the two areas, especially in the presence of surgical interventions of high complexity.

However, awareness of this correlation did not lead to consistent changes within the surgical community.

Indeed, adopting the policy of centralizing certain surgical procedures is far from trivial and involves a series of issues. These include logistical and organizational factors, which have a significant impact not only on healthcare organization but also on the lives of our patients and their families.

The monograph sets out to present an accurate state-of-the art picture of this controversial issue thanks to an up-to-date analysis of the literature and the use of data from the Ministry of Health and our Italian specialized government agency, the latter also contributing a specific chapter to the volume.

I would like to thank the many outstanding and experienced colleagues, who represent the majority of the leading specialist scientific societies in Italy, for their enthusiastic collaboration in the drafting of the various chapters on specific onco-logical diseases.

Essential to the debate are the chapters providing snapshot situations in the USA and in the rest of Europe, for which my gratitude is extended to my friend and Honorary Member of our Society Fabrizio Michelassi and to Pierre Alain Clavien at the European Surgical Association for the excellent collaboration.

The work is completed by a series of other more general chapters, which deal with some closely related organizational issues. One such chapter illustrates the processes which guarantee the correct measurement of surgical performance, its monitoring and its use, in the light of achieving an effective policy for the quality of healthcare services, a policy not yet so widespread in our country.

I am very proud to present the result of this long and complex collective work to the public and I believe that the monograph will contribute to the clarification of ideas and positions to be taken on this issue.

This joint effort has brought together the best of our surgical communities and national scientific societies and we hope that it will also prompt our institutions to officially consider the question in hand and activate effective regulatory action.

Milan, Italy   Marco Montorsi
September 2020

Contents

Contributors

Luca Alberti Division of General and Upper Gastrointestinal Surgery, Department of Surgery, Dentistry, Pediatrics and Gynecology, University of Verona, Verona, Italy

Marco Albini Quality Monitoring Office, Humanitas Clinical and Research Center IRCCS, Rozzano, Milan, Italy

Marco E. Allaix Department of Surgical Sciences, University of Turin, Turin, Italy

Grazia Maria Attinà Department of General Surgery, S. Camillo-Forlanini Hospital, Rome, Italy

Gianpaolo Balzano Division of Pancreatic Surgery, Pancreas Translational and Clinical Research Center, San Raffaele Scientific Institute, Milan, Italy

Claudio Bassi Department of General and Pancreatic Surgery, Pancreas Institute, University and Hospital Trust of Verona, G.B. Rossi Hospital, University of Verona, Verona, Italy

Rocco Bellantone Centro Dipartimentale di Chirurgia Endocrina e dell'Obesità, Fondazione Policlinico Universitario Agostino Gemelli IRCCS, Università Cattolica del Sacro Cuore, Rome, Italy

Francesco Bevere General Director's Office, Italian National Agency for Regional Healthcare Services, Rome, Italy

Paolo Pietro Bianchi Division of General and Minimally Invasive Surgery, Department of Surgery South-East Tuscany, Misericordia Hospital, Grosseto, Italy

Felice Borghi General and Oncologic Surgical Unit, Department of Surgery, Santa Croce e Carle Hospital, Cuneo, Italy

Lucia Borsellino Technical-Scientific Coordination, Italian National Agency for Regional Healthcare Services, Rome, Italy

Giulia Caraceni Pancreatic Surgery Unit, Humanitas Clinical and Research Center IRCCS, Rozzano, Milan, Italy

Rosetta Cardone Office for Review and Monitoring of Clinical Networks and Organizational Development, Italian National Agency for Regional Healthcare Services, Rome, Italy

Oriana Ciani Centre for Research for Health and Social Care Management—CERGAS, SDA Bocconi University, Milan, Italy

Pierre-Alain Clavien Department of Surgery and Transplantation, University Hospital Zurich, Zurich, Switzerland

Mimma Cosentino Office for Review and Monitoring of Clinical Networks and Organizational Development, Italian National Agency for Regional Healthcare Services, Rome, Italy

Carmela De Crea Centro Dipartimentale di Chirurgia Endocrina e dell'Obesità, Fondazione Policlinico Universitario Agostino Gemelli IRCCS, Università Cattolica del Sacro Cuore, Rome, Italy

Giovanni de Manzoni Division of General and Upper Gastrointestinal Surgery, Department of Surgery, Dentistry, Pediatrics and Gynecology, University of Verona, Verona, Italy

Carlo Alberto De Pasqual Division of General and Upper Gastrointestinal Surgery, Department of Surgery, Dentistry, Pediatrics and Gynecology, University of Verona, Verona, Italy

Giorgio De Toma Dipartimento di Chirurgia P. Valdoni, Sapienza University of Rome, Rome, Italy

Matteo Donadon Department of Biomedical Sciences, Humanitas University, Pieve Emanuele, Milan, Italy
Department of Hepatobiliary and General Surgery, Humanitas Clinical and Research Center IRCCS, Rozzano, Milan, Italy

Sofia Esposito Division of General, Emergency Surgery and New Technologies, Baggiovara General Hospital, Modena, Italy

Massimo Falconi Division of Pancreatic Surgery, Pancreas Translational and Clinical Research Center, San Raffaele Scientific Institute, Milan, Italy

Valeria Fava Cittadinanzattiva onlus, Rome, Italy

Giampaolo Formisano Division of General and Minimally Invasive Surgery, Department of Surgery South-East Tuscany, Misericordia Hospital, Grosseto, Italy

Eloisa Franchi Department of Hepatobiliary and General Surgery, Humanitas Clinical and Research Center IRCCS, Rozzano, Milan, Italy

Antonio Gaudioso Cittadinanzattiva onlus, Rome, Italy

Alessandro Ghirardini Office for Review and Monitoring of Clinical Networks and Organizational Development, Italian National Agency for Regional Healthcare Services, Rome, Italy

Simona Gorietti Office for Review and Monitoring of Clinical Networks and Organizational Development, Italian National Agency for Regional Healthcare Services, Rome, Italy

Alessandro Gronchi Sarcoma Service, Department of Surgery, Fondazione IRCCS Istituto Nazionale dei Tumori, Milan, Italy

Baldassare Ippolito Office for Review and Monitoring of Clinical Networks and Organizational Development, Italian National Agency for Regional Healthcare Services, Rome, Italy

Samuel Käser Department of Surgery and Transplantation, University Hospital Zurich, Zurich, Switzerland

Giorgio Leomporra Office for Review and Monitoring of Clinical Networks and Organizational Development, Italian National Agency for Regional Healthcare Services, Rome, Italy

Jason B. Liu Department of Surgery, University of Chicago Medicine, Chicago, IL, USA

Celestino Pio Lombardi Centro Dipartimentale di Chirurgia Endocrina e dell'Obesità, Fondazione Policlinico Universitario Agostino Gemelli IRCCS, Università Cattolica del Sacro Cuore, Rome, Italy,

Pierluigi Marini Department of General Surgery, S. Camillo-Forlanini Hospital, Rome, Italy

Emilia Marrazzo Breast Unit, Humanitas Clinical and Research Center IRCCS, Rozzano, Milan, Italy

Maria Grazia Marvulli Office for Review and Monitoring of Clinical Networks and Organizational Development, Italian National Agency for Regional Healthcare Services, Rome, Italy

Anna Maria Mele Department of Public Health and Infectious Diseases, Sapienza University of Rome, Rome, Italy

Patrizia Meroni Quality Management, Humanitas Clinical and Research Center IRCCS, Rozzano, Milan, Italy

Fabrizio Michelassi Department of Surgery, New York-Presbyterian Hospital at Weill Cornell, New York, NY, USA

Marco Montorsi Department of Biomedical Sciences, Humanitas University, Pieve Emanuele, Milan, Italy
Department of General Surgery, Humanitas Clinical and Research Center IRCCS, Rozzano, Milan, Italy

Mario Morino Department of Surgical Sciences, University of Turin, Turin, Italy

Barbara Mullineris Division of General, Emergency Surgery and New Technologies, Baggiovara General Hospital, Modena, Italy

Tiziana Nicoletti Cittadinanzattiva onlus, Rome, Italy

Francesco Pennestrì Centro Dipartimentale di Chirurgia Endocrina e dell'Obesità, Fondazione Policlinico Universitario Agostino Gemelli IRCCS, Università Cattolica del Sacro Cuore, Rome, Italy

Andrea Peri Department of Surgery, Fondazione IRCCS Policlinico San Matteo, Pavia, Italy

Micaela Piccoli Division of General, Emergency Surgery and New Technologies, Baggiovara General Hospital, Modena, Italy

Andrea Pietrabissa Department of Surgery, Fondazione IRCCS Policlinico San Matteo, University of Pavia, Pavia, Italy

Luigi Pugliese Department of Surgery, Fondazione IRCCS Policlinico San Matteo, Pavia, Italy

Vittorio Quagliuolo Department of Surgery, Humanitas Clinical and Research Center IRCCS, Rozzano, Milan, Italy

Marco Raffaelli Centro Dipartimentale di Chirurgia Endocrina e dell'Obesità, Fondazione Policlinico Universitario Agostino Gemelli IRCCS, Università Cattolica del Sacro Cuore Rome, Italy

Tecla Sansolini Office for Review and Monitoring of Clinical Networks and Organizational Development, Italian National Agency for Regional Healthcare Services, Rome, Italy

Claudio Seraschi Office for Review and Monitoring of Clinical Networks and Organizational Development, Italian National Agency for Regional Healthcare Services, Rome, Italy

Margherita Serra Breast Unit, Department of Woman, Child and Urological Diseases, Policlinico Sant'Orsola-Malpighi, University of Bologna, Bologna, Italy

Antonino Spinelli Department of Biomedical Sciences, Humanitas University, Pieve Emanuele, Milan, Italy
Colon and Rectal Surgery Division, Humanitas Clinical and Research Center IRCCS, Rozzano, Milan, Italy

Gaya Spolverato Department of Surgical, Oncological and Gastroenterological Sciences, University of Padua, Padua, Italy

Mario Taffurelli Breast Unit, Department of Woman, Child and Urological Diseases, Policlinico Sant'Orsola-Malpighi, University of Bologna, Bologna, Italy

Rosanna Tarricone Centre for Research for Health and Social Care Management—CERGAS, SDA Bocconi University, Milan, Italy
Department of Social and Political Science, Bocconi University, Milan, Italy

Mario Testini U.O.C. Chirurgia Generale Universitaria V. Bonomo, Università degli Studi di Bari Aldo Moro, A.O.U. Consorziale Policlinico di Bari, Bari, Italy

Corrado Tinterri Breast Unit, Humanitas Clinical and Research Center IRCCS, Rozzano, Milan, Italy

Aleksandra Torbica Centre for Research for Health and Social Care Management—CERGAS, SDA Bocconi University, Milan, Italy
Department of Social and Political Science, Bocconi University, Milan, Italy

Guido Torzilli Department of Biomedical Sciences, Humanitas University, Pieve Emanuele, Milan, Italy
Department of Hepatobiliary and General Surgery, Humanitas Clinical and Research Center IRCCS, Rozzano, Milan, Italy

Elena Vanni Business Operations, Humanitas Clinical and Research Center IRCCS, Rozzano, Milan, Italy

René Vonlanthen Department of Surgery and Transplantation, University Hospital Zurich, Zurich, Switzerland

Jacopo Weindelmayer Division of General and Upper Gastrointestinal Surgery, Department of Surgery, Dentistry, Pediatrics and Gynecology, University of Verona, Verona, Italy

Alessandro Zerbi Pancreatic Surgery Unit, Humanitas Clinical and Research Center IRCCS, Rozzano, Milan, Italy
Department of Biomedical Sciences, Humanitas University, Pieve Emanuele, Milan, Italy

The Relationship Between Volume and Outcome in Surgery: A Brief Introduction

1

Matteo Donadon and Marco Montorsi

1.1 Forty Years of Studies

The first report of the relationship between volume and outcome in surgery was that from Luft et al. in 1979 [1, 2], who showed higher mortality rates in patients who underwent complex procedures in low volume centers. Since then, many different original studies and systematic reviews have reported a positive relationship between hospital volume and clinical outcome for different surgical procedures [3–7]. In particular, Birkmeyer et al. [8, 9] have clearly shown how the quality and quantity of surgical operations were related, consistent with the slogan "the more I do, the better I do". Indeed, based on millions of operations, mostly on cancer patients, a positive correlation between 30-day mortality and number of operations was confirmed both for raw and for risk-adjusted data. This was found to be relevant mainly for high-risk procedures such as pancreatic and esophageal resections. These findings were recently validated by Morche et al. [10], who performed a systematic review of the subject. Among 32 reviews on 15 different high-risk procedures, the positive correlation between volume and outcome was confirmed, although methodological quality of most of the reviews analyzed was only moderate.

M. Donadon
Department of Biomedical Sciences, Humanitas University, Pieve Emanuele, Milan, Italy
Department of Hepatobiliary and General Surgery, Humanitas Clinical
and Research Center IRCCS, Rozzano, Milan, Italy
e-mail: matteo.donadon@hunimed.eu

M. Montorsi (✉)
Department of Biomedical Sciences, Humanitas University, Pieve Emanuele, Milan, Italy
Department of General Surgery, Humanitas Clinical and Research Center IRCCS, Rozzano, Milan, Italy
e-mail: marco.montorsi@hunimed.eu

© Springer Nature Switzerland AG 2021
M. Montorsi (ed.), *Volume-Outcome Relationship in Oncological Surgery*,
Updates in Surgery, https://doi.org/10.1007/978-3-030-51806-6_1

Starting from there, specific national policies have been implemented worldwide to centralize high-complexity procedures with the aim of improving the overall quality of care. Some successful European examples of these policies include those adopted in the United Kingdom, where the centralization of esophagogastric and pancreatic surgery has decreased mortality by 5% and 1%, respectively [11, 12], in Denmark, where there is a strong centralization with the highest rate of minimum number of cases per year [13], and in the Netherlands, where, similarly to the United Kingdom, the mortality rates after pancreatic resections significantly decreased from 9.8 to 3.6% [14]. However, these positive correlations between volume and outcome were found to be more evident for high-risk procedures only. Indeed, the same Dutch experience did not find any significant correlation between hospital volume and outcome after rectal surgery [15].

1.2   Some Open Questions

Despite the body of literature in favor of the volume-outcome relationship and of the consequent centralization of certain high-risk operations, many aspects require further investigation. Indeed, these volume-outcome analyses suffer some methodological limitations:

- the time perspective, which usually is limited to 30-day mortality;
- the volume cut-offs that have been reported almost arbitrarily in most of the published studies;
- the collinearity with other important determinants of hospital mortality, such as the so-called "failure to rescue", meaning that the decrease in mortality due to major complications is also dependent on the improvement of postoperative care, the quality of which is more closely related to some specific hospital characteristics (i.e., specialized intensive care unit, high nurse-to-patient ratios, etc.) than to the number of operations performed [16, 17];
- the conundrum of what is more important between surgeon volume and hospital volume, given that some operations require specific intraoperative skills (predominance of surgeon volume), and others may require major procedures during the postoperative course (predominance of hospital volume);
- the potential fallacy of extending the positive correlations between outcome and volume to low-risk procedures with a view to promoting centralization for personal/local interests.

It is important to note that there are some limitations to the centralization of surgical procedures.

- *First*, the increase in travel requirements of patients and relatives, which means increased costs for the patient's family and in general for society. Increased distance between home and hospital means prolonged waiting times, fragmentation of the continuity of care in the community, and exposure of the patients to inconveniences and risks that should not be neglected—especially in the case of aged patients. Very few studies have investigated the patient decision-making process, but Liu et al. [18] have shown that the driving distance likely remains the main reason why patients choose to undergo complex cancer operations at low-volume centers.

- *Second*, the training of specialized surgeons should be guaranteed throughout the country without restrictions. Thus, also complex surgical procedures should be available in high-quality centers across the country, and networking among the centers might be optimized to improve the quality of care.
- *Third*, it is interesting to note that the improved outcome in high-volume centers may follow two scenarios: outcome parameters may reach a plateau after a given cut-off number of procedures or may be associated with poorer results when a given hospital reaches its limit [19]. Considering that the number of hospital beds, specialized intensivists, specialized surgeons, and specialized nurses is finite, this second scenario is not so improbable in the real world.

While waiting for new studies on the subject, surgeons, clinicians and other health professionals will have to tackle these issues on their own so as to be active runners in this important match. Hospital volume acts as a proxy measure and/or surrogate of technical and non-technical elements that need to be identified and assessed in both low- and high-volume centers [20, 21].

The debate is thriving, and we gladly introduce this collection of contributions by outstanding and world-renowned authors in the hope of sustaining it with objective data and thoughts.

References

1. Luft HS, Bunker JP, Enthoven AC. Should operations be regionalized? The empirical relation between surgical volume and mortality. N Engl J Med. 1979;301(25):1364–9.
2. Luft HS. The relation between surgical volume and mortality: an exploration of causal factors and alternative models. Med Care. 1980;18(9):940–59.
3. Gruen RL, Pitt V, Green S, et al. The effect of provider case volume on cancer mortality: systematic review and meta-analysis. CA Cancer J Clin. 2009;59(3):192–211.
4. Finks JF, Osborne NH, Birkmeyer JD. Trends in hospital volume and operative mortality for high-risk surgery. N Engl J Med. 2011;364(22):2128–37.
5. Liu JH, Zingmond DS, McGory ML, et al. Disparities in the utilization of high-volume hospitals for complex surgery. JAMA. 2006;296(16):1973–80.
6. Pearse RM, Moreno RP, Bauer P, et al. Mortality after surgery in Europe: a 7 day cohort study. Lancet. 2012;380(9847):1059–65.
7. Bauer H, Honselmann KC. Minimum volume standards in surgery—are we there yet? Visc Med. 2017;33(2):106–16.
8. Birkmeyer JD, Siewers AE, Finlayson EV, et al. Hospital volume and surgical mortality in the United States. N Engl J Med. 2002;346(15):1128–37.
9. Birkmeyer JD, Stukel TA, Siewers AE, et al. Surgeon volume and operative mortality in the United States. N Engl J Med. 2003;349(2):2117–27.
10. Morche J, Mathes T, Pieper D. Relationship between surgeon volume and outcomes: a systematic review of systematic reviews. Syst Rev. 2016;5(1):204. https://doi.org/10.1186/s13643-016-0376-4.

11. Mole DJ, Parks RW. Centralization of surgery for pancreatic cancer. In: Shrikhande SV, Büchler MW, editors. Surgery of pancreatic cancer: current issues. New Delhi: Elsevier; 2012.
12. Varagunam M, Hardwick R, Riley S, et al. Changes in volume, clinical practice and outcome after reorganisation of oesophago-gastric cancer care in England: a longitudinal observational study. Eur J Surg Oncol. 2018;44(4):524–31.
13. Cronin-Fenton DP, Erichsen R, Mortensen FV, et al. Pancreatic cancer survival in central and northern Denmark from 1998 through 2009: a population-based cohort study. Clin Epidemiol. 2011;3(Suppl 1):19–25.
14. Mesman R, Faber MJ, Berden BJJM, Westert GP. Evaluation of minimum volume standards for surgery in the Netherlands (2003–2017): a successful policy? Health Policy. 2017;121(12):1263–73.
15. Jonker FHW, Hagemans JAW, Burger JWA, et al. The influence of hospital volume on long-term oncological outcome after rectal cancer surgery. Int J Color Dis. 2017;32(12):1741–7.
16. Spolverato G, Ejaz A, Hyder O, et al. Failure to rescue as a source of variation in hospital mortality after hepatic surgery. Br J Surg. 2014;101(7):836–46.
17. Buettner S, Gani F, Amini N, et al. The relative effect of hospital and surgeon volume on failure to rescue among patients undergoing liver resection for cancer. Surgery. 2016;159(4):1004–12.
18. Liu JB, Bilimoria KY, Mallin K, Winchester DP. Patient characteristics associated with undergoing cancer operations at low-volume hospitals. Surgery. 2017;161(2):433–43.
19. Vonlanthen R, Lodge P, Barkun JS, et al. Toward a consensus on centralization in surgery. Ann Surg. 2018;268(5):712–24.
20. Mesman R, Faber MJ, Westert GP, Berden HJJM. Dutch surgeons' views on the volume-outcome mechanism in surgery: a qualitative interview study. Int J Qual Health Care. 2017;29(6):797–802.
21. Ravaioli M, Pinna AD, Francioni G, et al. A partnership model between high- and low-volume hospitals to improve results in hepatobiliary pancreatic surgery. Ann Surg. 2014;260(5):871–5; discussion 875–7.

Core Outcome Set in Surgical Oncology: Why, What and How to Measure

2

Oriana Ciani, Aleksandra Torbica, and Rosanna Tarricone

2.1 Introduction

The establishment of the evidence-based medicine paradigm has promoted the use of clinical trials to evaluate whether interventions are effective and safe for patients by comparing their relative effects on outcomes chosen to identify benefits and harms. Careful selection of outcome measures is essential if research and audit is to inform clinical practice and guide health policy, as decision makers, clinical professionals and patients use this information to make well-informed healthcare choices.

However, recent studies have demonstrated a largely inconsistent approach to the selection, definition, measurement and reporting of outcomes. Inadequate attention to the choice of outcomes in clinical trials has led to avoidable waste in the production and reporting of research, as the outcomes considered are not always those regarded as most important or relevant by key stakeholders (patients, decision-makers, health professionals) [1]. The outcomes may also be differently defined and measured, thus making it difficult or impossible to synthesize the results of different research studies in a meta-analysis and apply them in a meaningful way to inform practice.

O. Ciani
Centre for Research for Health and Social Care Management—CERGAS, SDA Bocconi University, Milan, Italy
e-mail: oriana.ciani@unibocconi.it

A. Torbica · R. Tarricone (✉)
Centre for Research for Health and Social Care Management—CERGAS, SDA Bocconi University, Milan, Italy
Department of Social and Political Science, Bocconi University, Milan, Italy
e-mail: aleksandra.torbica@unibocconi.it; rosanna.tarricone@unibocconi.it

© Springer Nature Switzerland AG 2021
M. Montorsi (ed.), *Volume-Outcome Relationship in Oncological Surgery*,
Updates in Surgery, https://doi.org/10.1007/978-3-030-51806-6_2

2.2   Core Outcome Measures in Surgical Oncology: Why?

A systematic analysis of oncology research found that more than 25,000 outcomes had appeared only once or twice in oncology trials [2]. Out of 134 clinical studies in reconstructive breast surgery, less than 20% of the 950 outcomes assessed were clearly defined, with lack of consistency across definitions based on timing of occurrence, method of diagnosis, mode of treatment [3].

Alongside inconsistency in the measurement of outcomes, opportunities for outcome reporting bias exist and add to the problems faced by people trying to use healthcare research.

There is a clear need for consistent and appropriate selection, measurement, use and reporting of outcomes in clinical research and practice. The inconsistencies and bias due to incomparable data available on the effects of interventions could be addressed with the development and application of agreed standardized sets of outcomes, known as core outcome sets (COS), to be measured and reported as a minimum requirement in all effectiveness trials for a specific health area. Effective implementation of COS ensures that all trials provide usable evidence, allows cross-study comparisons and may inform data collection and discussion during clinical encounters. COS are not intended to restrict the number of outcomes in a particular trial; rather, the intention is to set out the basic outcomes that will always be collected and reported, whilst investigators are fully expected to continue to explore additional outcomes [4].

2.3   Core Outcome Set in Surgical Oncology: What?

A COS may be developed to cover all aspects of a disease or health condition, but it may also focus on a particular type of treatment only, or on a specific age group or stage of disease. According to a recent taxonomy for outcome classification, outcomes included in core sets can be classified in a variety of domains from survival/mortality to physiological or clinical, adverse events, functioning, delivery of care, global quality of life, personal circumstances and resource use [5]. In many cases these outcomes are assessed as patient-reported outcomes (PROs). PROs can be defined as a measurement of any aspect of a patient's health status that comes directly from the patient, without the interpretation of the patient's responses by a physician or anyone else [6].

The Outcomes Measures in Rheumatoid Arthritis Clinical Trials (OMERACT) initiative led a pioneering development of a COS in rheumatoid arthritis, followed by similar efforts in other disease areas [7]. The International Consortium for Health Outcomes Measurement (ICHOM) has published, up to March 2020, 32 standard sets which are standardized outcomes, measurement tools and time points and risk-adjustment factors covering different conditions and specific patient populations (https://www.ichom.org/standard-sets/). The COMET (Core Outcome Measures in Effectiveness Trials) initiative aims to collate and stimulate the development, application and promotion of COS, by supplying relevant resources and methodological support. One of such resources is the COMET database, a publicly available internet-based platform that includes published accounts of COS development, as well as planned and ongoing work [8].

Latest reports on the COMET database reveal that oncology is the most prevalent disease category (16%) among included studies, and surgery is the focus of 8% of entries [4]. These studies originated predominantly in North America (83%) and Europe (76%). The implications of this research go beyond the clinical trialists' community, as the developers of 11% of the COS identified intended their recommendations for clinical practice as well as health research.

As of September 2019, among the 250 entries in the COMET database, we identified 8 studies defining relevant outcome sets in surgical oncology according to the content of this handbook: two in gastric cancer [9, 10], two in esophageal cancer [11, 12], one in breast cancer (reconstructive breast surgery) [13], and three in colorectal cancer [14–16] (Table 2.1). Four ongoing and still unpublished studies in pancreatic cancer (http://www.comet-initiative.org/studies/details/280), liver cancer (http://www.comet-initiative.org/studies/details/607), lung cancer (http://www.comet-initiative.org/studies/details/659) and emergency surgery (http://www.comet-initiative.org/studies/details/1099) were excluded, as well as two commentaries [17, 18] and a patient perspective report from the BRAVO (Breast Reconstruction and Valid Outcomes) study [19], whose main output has been included in our analysis.

The stakeholder groups involved in developing a COS vary between clinical areas. Whilst two studies do not involve stakeholders other than the reviewers writing the report, there has been a trend towards greater involvement of patient and public representatives (also caregivers, patient support groups and charities), which are included in 59% of all COS identified by COMET [4]. Clinical experts continue to be involved in almost all studies and sometimes manufacturers, epidemiologists and investigators are consulted.

The methods applied range from systematic reviews of clinical studies to comprehensively identify a list of outcomes for a health condition to face-to-face interviews and structured methods for consensus generation (e.g., consensus meeting, Delphi process, nominal group technique).

Tables 2.2, 2.3, 2.4, and 2.5 provide a summary of the relevant outcomes recommended by the different studies for inclusion in COS across disease categories.

These outcomes are generally classified as mortality/survival measures (e.g., in-hospital, perioperative, long-term), adverse events and complications (e.g., anastomotic leak), symptoms (e.g., diarrhea, nausea), delivery of care and resource use (e.g., length of stay, operation time), quality of life (e.g., role function, social function).

Two of the studies focus specifically on PROs and patient-reported outcome measures (PROMs) to be included in COS for colorectal and gastric cancer, respectively. Challenges in the identification and selection of relevant PROs in COS are accentuated by the abundance of different (and often ill-defined) questionnaires, the multiplicity of items and scales per questionnaire and lack of a universally agreed terminology [20].

Table 2.1 Main characteristics of core outcome set (COS) studies in surgical oncology

First author	Year	Disease categories	Disease name/ type of intervention	Sex	Method(s)	Stakeholders involved	Study type
Alkhaffaf [9]	2018	Gastric cancer	Cancer, Gastroenterology /Surgery	Either	Systematic review	None	[a] Systematic review of outcomes measured in trials
Avery [11]	2017	Esophageal cancer	Cancer/Surgery	Either	Consensus meeting; Delphi process; Systematic review; Interview	Consumers (patients); Clinical experts	COS for clinical trials or clinical research
McNair [15]	2016	Colorectal cancer	Cancer/Surgery	Either	Consensus meeting; Delphi process; Systematic review; Interview; Nominal group technique (NGT)	Consumers (patients); Clinical experts; Consumers (caregivers)	COS for clinical trials or clinical research
Potter [13]	2015	Reconstructive breast surgery	Other/Surgery	Female	Consensus meeting; Delphi process; Systematic review; Interview	Consumers (patients); Clinical experts; Charities; Patient/ support group representatives; Device manufacturers	COS for clinical trials or clinical research
Blazeby [12]	2015	Esophageal cancer	Cancer/Surgery	Either	Consensus meeting; Delphi process; Literature review	Consumers (patients); Clinical experts	Core information set
McNair [14]	2015	Colorectal cancer	Cancer/Surgery	Either	Systematic review	Study investigators	[a] Systematic review of outcomes measured in trials; Systematic review of outcome measures/ measurement instruments
Whistance [16]	2013	Colorectal cancer	Cancer/Surgery	Either	Systematic review	None	[a] Systematic review of outcomes measured in trials
Karanicolas [10]	2011	Gastric cancer	Cancer, Gastroenterology /Surgery	Either	Systematic review	Clinical experts; Epidemiologists	Overview of literature

[a]First stage of studies that aim to define COS and reach consensus on the most important outcomes amongst key stakeholders

Table 2.2 Core outcome sets proposed in surgical oncology—colorectal cancer

Whistance 2013 [16]	McNair 2015 [14][a]	McNair 2016 [15]
• Overall survival, 30-day mortality, postoperative mortality • Anastomotic leak, wound infection • Local recurrence, distant recurrence • Number of retrieved lymph nodes, circumferential resection margin • Diarrhea, nausea • Operation time, blood loss • Reoperation, hospital stay, hospital readmission	• Bodily pain • General health perceptions • Mental health • Physical functioning • Role limitations due to emotional health problems • Role limitations due to physical health problems • Social functioning • Vitality [Short Form 36 (SF-36), generic] • Physical domain • Role domain • Emotional domain • Social domain • Cognitive domain • Global health status • Fatigue • Pain • Emesis • Further symptoms [EORTC Quality of life questionnaire (QLQ-C30), cancer-specific] • Body image • Sexual function • Micturition problems • Gastrointestinal tract symptoms • Chemotherapy side effects • Defecation problems • Stoma-related problems • Sexual problems • Sexual enjoyment • Weight loss • Future perspective [EORTC Colorectal Cancer Module (QLQ-CR38), disease-specific]	• Long-term survival • Cancer recurrence • Resection margins • Anastomotic leak • Perioperative survival • Surgical site infection • Stoma rates and complications • Conversion to open operation (where appropriate) • Physical function • Sexual function • Fecal incontinence • Fecal urgency

EORTC European Organisation for Research and Treatment of Cancer
[a]Study specifically dealing with patient-reported outcome measures (PROs) and patient-reported outcome measures (PROMs) to be included in core outcome sets

Table 2.3 Core outcome sets proposed in surgical oncology—gastric cancer

Karanicolas 2011 [10][a]	Alkhaffaf 2018 [9]
• Dysphagia • Pain • Reflux • Eating • Anxiety • Taste • Hair loss • Dry mouth • Body image [EORTC Stomach Module (STO-22)] • Core symptoms • Physical items • Psychological items • Social items • Disease-specific [Gastrointestinal Quality of Life Index (GIQLI)] • Reflux • Abdominal pain • Indigestion • Diarrhea • Constipation [Gastrointestinal Symptom Rating Scale (GSRS)]	• 5-year survival • Number of lymph nodes dissected/resected/retrieved • Operative time • Pancreatic fistula • Duration of hospital stay • Duration of postoperative hospital stay • Pneumonia • Wound infection • Abdominal abscess

EORTC European Organisation for Research and Treatment of Cancer
[a]Study specifically dealing with patient-reported outcomes (PROs) and patient-reported outcome measures (PROMs) to be included in core outcome sets

Table 2.4 Core outcome sets proposed in surgical oncology—esophageal cancer

Avery 2017 [11]	Blazeby 2015 [12]
• Overall survival • In-hospital mortality • Inoperability • The need for another operation related to their primary esophageal cancer resection surgery • Respiratory complications • Conduit necrosis and anastomotic leak • Severe nutritional problems • Ability to eat and drink • Problems with acid indigestion or heartburn • Overall quality of life	• Expected in-hospital experiences and milestones to recovery (including length of stay and pain control) • Chances of inoperability • Information about major complications (reoperation, leak, respiratory problems) • In-hospital mortality • Expected recovery milestones after discharge and follow-up • Impact on eating and drinking in the longer term • Long-term overall quality of life • Long-term survival

Table 2.5 Core outcome set proposed in surgical oncology—reconstructive breast surgery

Potter 2015 [13]

- Implant-related complications[a]
- Flap-related complications[a]
- Major complications[b] leading to readmission to hospital
- Unplanned surgery for any reason[b]
- Donor-site problems/morbidity[b]
- Self-esteem[c]
- Emotional well-being[c]
- Normality[b] Feeling "back to normal self"
- Quality of life[b]
- Physical well-being[c]
- Women's cosmetic satisfaction[b]

[a]Item core to professional group only
[b]Item core to both patients and professionals
[c]Item core to patient group only

2.4   Core Outcome Set in Surgical Oncology: How to Measure?

The first step in COS development is typically 'what to measure', which is the domain necessary to measure and report in health research or clinical practice. Recommendations on 'when' and 'how', what outcome measurement instruments (OMIs) to use, usually follow. Gargon et al. estimated that about 38% of COS studies contained recommendations about how to measure the outcomes in the COS [1]. In this respect, the Consensus-based Standards for the selection of health Measurement Instruments (COSMIN) initiative is to be referenced (http://www.cosmin.nl/). COSMIN aims to improve the selection of OMIs, and has developed methodological standards for studies on the measurement properties of OMIs. In the evaluation of the measurement properties of the OMIs that could potentially be included in a COS, COSMIN recommends a predefined order of importance:

1. content validity;
2. internal structure (i.e., structural validity and internal consistency, and/or Item Response Theory (IRT)/Rasch model fit);
3. where applicable, the remaining measurement properties (i.e., reliability, measurement error, hypotheses testing, cross-cultural validity, criterion validity, and responsiveness) [21].

2.5   Conclusions

In this chapter we have illustrated some examples of COS proposed for relevant surgical oncology specialties. The selection of appropriate outcomes in clinical research needs greater attention from the scientific community, if findings are to be easily translated to practice and useful, reliable, and relevant to patients, healthcare professionals, and others making decisions regarding healthcare provision. Overall, effectiveness trials, being more or less pragmatic, are designed to assess whether an intervention is effective for routine clinical practice and outcomes, therefore, need to be relevant and important to patients as well as clinicians and other key decision-makers. The involvement of the public in the development of COS is particularly relevant for comparative effectiveness research, where long-term patient-centered outcomes are often the important endpoints. The types of people who are regarded as (or determined to be) key to developing a COS are likely to involve clinical experts and the public.

It is of paramount importance for health information systems today to be able to collect, record and interpret the outcomes recommended for measurement in COS, including PROMs [22], which have been traditionally neglected by the clinical and performance data records. The advent and fast development of mobile health technologies will certainly foster the process.

References

1. Gargon E, Gurung B, Medley N, et al. Choosing important health outcomes for comparative effectiveness research: a systematic review. PLoS One. 2014;9(6):e99111. https://doi.org/10.1371/journal.pone.0099111.
2. Hirsch BR, Califf RM, Cheng SK, et al. Characteristics of oncology clinical trials: insights from a systematic analysis of ClinicalTrials.gov. JAMA Intern Med. 2013;173(11):972–9.
3. Potter S, Brigic A, Whiting PF, et al. Reporting clinical outcomes of breast reconstruction: a systematic review. J Natl Cancer Inst. 2011;103(1):31–46.
4. Gorst SL, Gargon E, Clarke M, et al. Choosing important health outcomes for comparative effectiveness research: an updated review and identification of gaps. PLoS One. 2016;11(12):e0168403. https://doi.org/10.1371/journal.pone.0168403.
5. Dodd S, Clarke M, Becker L, et al. A taxonomy has been developed for outcomes in medical research to help improve knowledge discovery. J Clin Epidemiol. 2018;96:84–92.
6. Black N. Patient reported outcome measures could help transform healthcare. BMJ. 2013;346:f167. https://doi.org/10.1136/bmj.f167.
7. Tugwell P, Boers M, Brooks P, et al. OMERACT: an international initiative to improve outcome measurement in rheumatology. Trials. 2007;8:38. https://doi.org/10.1186/1745-6215-8-38.
8. Gargon E, Williamson PR, Altman DG, et al. The COMET initiative database: progress and activities update (2015). Trials. 2017;18(1):54. https://doi.org/10.1186/s13063-017-1788-8.
9. Alkhaffaf B, Blazeby JM, Williamson PR, et al. Reporting of outcomes in gastric cancer surgery trials: a systematic review. BMJ Open. 2018;8(10):e021796. https://doi.org/10.1136/bmjopen-2018-021796.
10. Karanicolas PJ, Bickenbach K, Jayaraman S, et al. Measurement and interpretation of patient-reported outcomes in surgery: an opportunity for improvement. J Gastrointest Surg. 2011;15(4):682–9.
11. Avery KNL, Chalmers KA, Brookes ST, et al. Development of a core outcome set for clinical effectiveness trials in esophageal cancer resection surgery. Ann Surg. 2018;267(4):700–10.
12. Blazeby JM, Macefield R, Blencowe NS, et al. Core information set for oesophageal cancer surgery. Br J Surg. 2015;102(8):936–43.
13. Potter S, Holcombe C, Ward JA, et al. Development of a core outcome set for research and audit studies in reconstructive breast surgery. Br J Surg. 2015;102(11):1360–71.

14. McNair AG, Whistance RN, Forsythe RO, et al. Synthesis and summary of patient-reported outcome measures to inform the development of a core outcome set in colorectal cancer surgery. Color Dis. 2015;17(11):O217–29.
15. McNair AG, Whistance RN, Forsythe RO, et al. Core outcomes for colorectal cancer surgery: a consensus study. PLoS Med. 2016;13(8):e1002071. https://doi.org/10.1371/journal.pmed.1002071.
16. Whistance RN, Forsythe RO, McNair AG, et al. A systematic review of outcome reporting in colorectal cancer surgery. Color Dis. 2013;15(10):e548–60.
17. Ward JA, Potter S, Blazeby JM. Outcome reporting for reconstructive breast surgery: the need for consensus, consistency and core outcome sets. Eur J Surg Oncol. 2012;38(11):1020–1.
18. Whistance RN, Blencowe NS, Blazeby JM. The need for standardised outcome reporting in colorectal surgery. Gut. 2012;61(3):472.
19. Potter S, Brookes ST, Holcombe C, et al. Exploring methods for the selection and integration of stakeholder views in the development of core outcome sets: a case study in reconstructive breast surgery. Trials. 2016;17(1):463. https://doi.org/10.1186/s13063-016-1591-y.
20. Macefield RC, Jacobs M, Korfage IJ, et al. Developing core outcomes sets: methods for identifying and including patient-reported outcomes (PROs). Trials. 2014;15:49. https://doi.org/10.1186/1745-6215-15-49.
21. Prinsen CA, Vohra S, Rose MR, et al. How to select outcome measurement instruments for outcomes included in a "Core Outcome Set"—a practical guideline. Trials. 2016;17(1):449. https://doi.org/10.1186/s13063-016-1555-2.
22. Meregaglia M, Ciani O, Banks H, et al. A scoping review of core outcome sets and their 'mapping' onto real-world data using prostate cancer as a case study. BMC Med Res Methodol. 2020;20(1):41. https://doi.org/10.1186/s12874-020-00928-w.

Role of AGENAS in the Development of Oncological Networks in Italy

3

Alessandro Ghirardini, Baldassare Ippolito,
Anna Maria Mele, Giorgio Leomporra, Rosetta Cardone,
Mimma Cosentino, Maria Grazia Marvulli, Simona Gorietti,
Claudio Seraschi, Tecla Sansolini, Lucia Borsellino,
and Francesco Bevere

3.1 Introduction

National healthcare services are undoubtedly facing complex challenges that require the formulation of care models increasingly oriented towards the integration of health services among the different supply areas, at either the hospital or community level. Various tools are currently available to foster this integration: in particular, the management of healthcare through the use of clinical networks is the main contributor to the modernization of the sector [1]. The last few years have been characterized by a progressive reduction in the spread of infectious diseases (the leading cause of death throughout past centuries) and the increase of chronically degenerative conditions together with an increasingly fragile healthcare service.

A. Ghirardini (✉) · B. Ippolito · G. Leomporra · R. Cardone
M. Cosentino · M. G. Marvulli · S. Gorietti · C. Seraschi · T. Sansolini
Office for Review and Monitoring of Clinical Networks and Organizational Development,
Italian National Agency for Regional Healthcare Services, Rome, Italy
e-mail: ghirardini@agenas.it; ippolito@agenas.it; leomporra@agenas.it;
r.cardone@sanita.it; cosentino@agenas.it; marvulli@agenas.it;
gorietti@agenas.it; seraschi@agenas.it; sansolini@agenas.it

A. M. Mele
Department of Public Health and Infectious Diseases,
Sapienza University of Rome, Rome, Italy
e-mail: annamaria.mele@uniroma1.it

L. Borsellino
Technical-Scientific Coordination, Italian National Agency
for Regional Healthcare Services, Rome, Italy
e-mail: borsellino@agenas.it

F. Bevere
General Director's Office, Italian National Agency
for Regional Healthcare Services, Rome, Italy
e-mail: dir@agenas.it

© Springer Nature Switzerland AG 2021   15
M. Montorsi (ed.), *Volume-Outcome Relationship in Oncological Surgery*,
Updates in Surgery, https://doi.org/10.1007/978-3-030-51806-6_3

In this peculiar framework, one cannot ignore the changing demographic scenario, characterized by the dramatic fall of births, the constant lengthening of life expectancy, the overall ageing of the population and, finally, the growth of immigration. In this perspective, the issue of oncological networks gains importance.

3.2 Background

The recent debate is rather controversial: on the one hand, oncological networks may help to overcome the asynchrony of their effective implementation at the national level; on the other, the still too limited presence of actual clinical networks for oncological patients cannot be disregarded. Despite the debate calling for the creation of oncological networks, only few Italian Regions have launched systematic programs for their creation. Within this context, the availability of different clinical and management models for oncological networks across the country should be regarded as an opportunity to valorize each experience and good practice in the field of oncology and applied research by spreading the existing know-how [2]. Considering the urgency of recognizing the value of oncological networks and their role in providing patients with high-quality care, serious strategic planning is needed together with an appropriate control and evaluation system. Future objectives should be appropriately specified through the extensive involvement of professionals, patients and institutions [3].

Among national regulations, specific mention of the objectives of networks is made in the National Health Plan (NHP) 2006–2008, whereas the following NHPs (2010–2012 and 2014–2016) mainly support the efficacy of cancer treatments by developing specific healthcare solutions which, through planning acts, back the principle of the development and implementation of hospital networks and healthcare integrated pathways (Italian PDTA, percorsi diagnostico terapeutici assistenziali) as fundamental fulfilments of the NHP.

Following the mandate received from the State-Regions Unified Conference in September 2007 with regard to hospital networks, the National Agency for Regional Healthcare Services (AGENAS) together with the Ministry of Health, the Regions and patients' associations promoted a debate to support the planning, implementation and quality assessment of management models for oncological networks and clinical pathways in oncology.

From a legal viewpoint, the task of establishing an Institutional Round Table and providing technical and scientific coordination in the area of both oncological and clinical networks has been assigned to AGENAS, which will formulate new guidelines and recommendations and update the existing ones, within the terms of the relevant regulation.

3.3 Methods

The Institutional Round Table has adopted a scheme recording clinical networks, as a joint monitoring tool, which includes the requirements of common reference for each clinical network, supported by current scientific and legal publications as well as relevant regulations.

The objective underpinning the methodology used for reviewing the organizational guidelines and oncological networks' recommendations, is to systematize the procedures, information and indicators at the disposal of each level of health governance in order to smooth the way for regular assessment and self-assessment.

The scheme identifies the basic common requirements of each oncological network that help to guarantee its effectiveness by ensuring the correct monitoring of planning and related management issues.

AGENAS—in collaboration with the relevant institutional players, such as the Ministry of Health, the Regions and the Autonomous Provinces of Trento and Bolzano, the National Institute of Public Health (ISS), the Italian Medicines Agency (AIFA), as well as healthcare experts, scientific societies, and the Cittadinanzattiva (Active Citizenship) association – has drafted a document including the review of the organizational guidelines and recommendations for oncological networks. The complex process of systematization of available experiences and good practices has required a well-structured working process: 13 technical workgroups (involving more than 200 professionals) working on advice of the Institutional Round Table and its Technical-Scientific Coordination (Fig. 3.1).

On April 17, 2019 the organizational guidelines and recommendations for the oncological hospital-community network were agreed on by Italian State-Regions Conference. The agreement recognizes the oncological network as the "keystone for healthcare continuity between the hospital and the community"; it is an organizational model which envisages a multidisciplinary approach for the clinical management of patients, sharing of care pathways and guaranteeing equity of access and prompt taking charge of patients [4].

The Agreement regarding oncological networks comprises ten lines of action that constitute a program of measures for the governance of oncological networks aiming to promote and enhance quality, security and appropriateness of health interventions in oncology. Given the complementarity of those lines of action, they require joint implementation at the national or regional and local level (Table 3.1).

The strategic value of the tasks carried out highlights the central role played by AGENAS, in collaboration with the Ministry of Health, the Regions and the Autonomous Provinces, in suggesting models and tools for monitoring and evaluating the implementation of regional oncological networks with the specific aim of guaranteeing solid technical-scientific support to Regions and Autonomous Provinces throughout the realization and evaluation of regional oncological networks and clinical pathways in oncology.

Fig. 3.1 Methodology followed to review the organizational guidelines of oncology

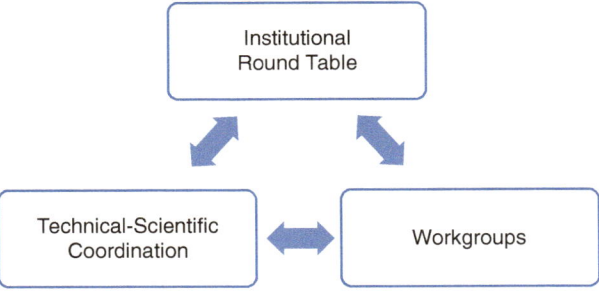

Table 3.1 Minimum
requirements for the
implementation and
functioning of a typical
oncological network

1. Health policy measures employable in governance
2. Allocation of resources
3. Operational mechanisms
4. Research at the network level
5. Education at the network level
6. Medicines
7. Social processes and support to people and care givers
8. Communication and transparency
9. Indicators
10. Monitoring and updating functions

3.4   Observatory on Oncological Networks

Section 10 of the Agreement between the State and the Regions of April 17, 2019 introduced a coordination system led by the Ministry of Health and provided for the establishment of an oncological network observatory, with the aim of improving the quality of care in oncology through the development of a permanent system for monitoring and evaluating the implementation of oncological networks [5]. This strategic coordination system, led by the Ministry of Health, will avail itself of an Observatory set up within AGENAS for the analysis, measurement and evaluation of the state of implementation of the directions in the regional contexts.

The Observatory on the monitoring and evaluation of oncological networks will assess the developments achieved and any persisting deficiency, providing citizens with a source of continuously updated and transparent data. Furthermore, the oncological network Observatory intends to serve as a connection and provide decision-making support in developing the oncological network strategies, in line with decisions agreed-upon by the Ministry of Health and the Regions; in this respect, the Observatory supports the process of consultation and facilitates information sharing.

The role of the Observatory involves study, research and data analysis; it also entails an operational and proactive function with reference to the decision-making and governance processes of the oncological networks. In addition to monitoring and evaluation, the functions of the Observatory also include technical consultancy (operative consultancy at the local and regional level for the solution of critical issues), innovation and training, dissemination and accountability, promotion of policies (in close cooperation with the Ministry of Health, in accordance with the institutional roles).

Its main activities are described in the following section.

3.4.1   Technical Support of the National Monitoring Processes

The Observatory on oncological networks supports the regions in monitoring of the implementation of the national oncological networks. Accordingly, it provides technical-operational assistance to the monitoring activities of the oncological networks. More specifically, the Observatory implements a specific system for the monitoring, analysis and control of the trends of the individual regional oncological networks, which, through a specific alert system, helps to preemptively detect any significant deviations in the performance of the different network facilities, in terms of appropriateness, equity and quality of the services provided.

In order to provide technical and operational assistance, the Observatory is supported by the AGENAS Office for review and monitoring of clinical networks and organizational development.

The aim of the monitoring process is to verify if the oncological networks can guarantee fair care settings and to provide general suggestions for service planning and organization, with the aim of improving the entire care pathway and ensuring continuity of care, appropriateness and quality. To this end, the Observatory promotes initiatives for research, exchange and action, with the aim of supporting the implementation and development of the oncological networks. In this respect, attention is given to the continuous improvement of the quality of clinical care pathways and to the full integration of services for oncology, particularly in terms of continuity of care.

3.4.2   Technical-Scientific Support to Regional Representatives/ Coordinators of Oncological Networks

This activity refers to the need to ensure that regional representatives properly enter data and information in the relevant fields of the online database by providing a helpdesk to assist with potential technical problems.

The Observatory, for the national monitoring process, establishes the timing, modalities and periodicity of the data collection, taking into consideration data that are collected and validated by the regional representatives within the established monitoring period. The Regions and Autonomous Provinces monitor the implementation of the regional oncological networks, and through the same instruments the Observatory performs semiannual monitoring.

3.4.3   Development of Periodic Reports

The main result of the Observatory is a periodic report mainly deals focusing on the institutionalization of the regional oncological networks and their activities.

The Observatory produces annual reports illustrating all the changes and characteristics of the phenomenon analyzed, promoting in-depth analysis of critical issues, and drafting the relative documentation.

The Observatory ensures that data and documents are constantly up-to-date, comparable, and telematically accessible. Moreover, it promotes meetings, discussions and training courses.

Reports produced by the Observatory include:

- quantitative and qualitative analysis of macro-variables related to the organizational model and governance system;
- analysis of activity/issues regarding human resources;
- descriptive and qualitative analysis of technical equipment;
- analysis of activities concerning funding and economic resources;
- analysis of patient pathways and related clinical pathways (PDTA);
- clinical and organizational research;
- analysis of the ability of regional oncological networks to provide training and updating courses to experts working for these networks;
- descriptive and qualitative analysis of the information technology system;
- analysis of the means of communication and transparency;
- analysis of the level of knowledge and competencies of workers involved in these networks;
- analysis of the knowledge and experience of patients, users and citizens;
- analysis and development of specific indicators for the evaluation of clinical, economic and organizational performances.

3.4.4   Contribution to the Development of Guidelines and Recommendations on Specific Matters, to Support Regions and Local Health Authorities

The current legislation requires AGENAS to achieve specific strategic objectives, including supporting the regions, disseminating at regional level the results of studies and assessments performed at central level, and promoting actions in line with these results.

In this legislative framework, the Observatory aims to help spread the innovations already introduced in clinical practice, by promoting actions and instruments to disseminate the recommendations, increase the circulation of information and foster the transfer of experience.

The Observatory on oncological networks helps to disseminate guidelines and recommendations. The different aspects of technological and organizational innovation and regional experiments are analyzed in order to suggest solutions to increase the efficiency and quality of health services and propose instruments to perform different governance activities, including direction, programming, assessment and control.

Innovating and experimenting are therefore key to developing an increasingly efficient healthcare system and responding to the needs of the population.

3.4.5   Promotion of the Implementation of Organizational Models and Innovating Programs for Healthcare in Oncology

The Observatory on oncological networks promotes the development of organizational models and innovative healthcare programs aimed at optimizing the integration of oncological rehabilitation and palliative care pathways based on the needs of patients, the creation of regional networks and the overall care system taking charge of all aspects of a patient's care.

The activities of the Observatory are characterized by the effective collaboration between oncological scientific societies, patient associations, universities and foundations, as well as Regions and the Government to discuss and exchange skills and expertise, in order to increase the quality of clinical care pathways.

The specific objectives of the project are:

- identifying quality standards in oncology with the collaboration of scientific societies;
- defining operational criteria for structuring and sizing community services for care and rehabilitation;
- experimenting and investigating the attitudes and perceptions of the subjects involved—professionals, caregivers and patients—as regards the organizational models for taking charge of the patients at different times of the clinical care pathway (communication of diagnosis, management of treatment and follow-up care, and integration of conventional and palliative therapies).

3.4.6   Promotion of Clinical Governance Models with the Involvement of Stakeholders

The activities of the Observatory are aimed at illustrating the potential of the network as: a clinical governance tool to support the appropriateness of care and continuity of care; a vehicle for promoting clinical research and training, and; a tool for sharing decisions and, above all, for the continuous improvement of the quality of healthcare, in terms of clinical efficacy and cost-effectiveness.

The Observatory aims to identify the innovative mechanisms of the network organization for the benefit of the patient in order to facilitate access to healthcare facilities and improve their quality, by promoting transparency in the offer and sustainability of the services.

3.4.7 Organizational Guidelines and Recommendations for the Improvement of Quality and Safety in the Oncological Networks and Pathways

In the national context, an organized and well-structured system for the update, review and implementation of the guidelines is necessary. The objective is to provide National Healthcare Service professionals with clinical and organizational guidance, in a consistent manner throughout the national territory.

Guidelines, as the other tools providing recommendations on clinical care and healthcare, are developed with the aim of guiding the decisions of medical professionals, also with the involvement of the patients, towards the most appropriate care for the most common diseases.

The Observatory intends to systematize the collection, processing, implementation and periodic review of the organizational guidelines and recommendations, and to foster the circulation of good practices. This will require the accurate definition of procedures and areas of intervention, which constitute the basis of the management of care pathways, safety in healthcare, and homogeneity of treatments, based on the diseases and care settings. The development of new organizational guidelines and the updating of existing ones allow us to take into consideration scientific and technological evolution and ensures more adequate, safe and appropriate care pathways for the patients, in response to the changes in health needs and technological and therapeutic innovations.

In line with the above, Fig. 3.2 shows the organizational model of the institutional functions carried out by the Observatory. In particular, the figure defines the activities behind the leading goal of the Observatory, and helps to understand the complex work done in different areas: monitoring, promotion, innovation, and dissemination.

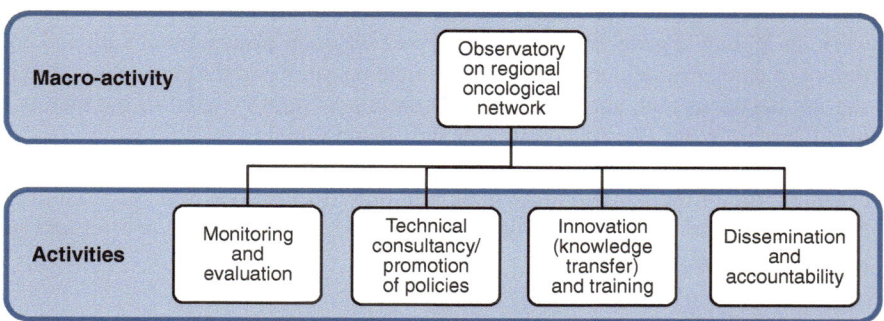

Fig. 3.2 Distribution of the main activities of the Observatory on regional oncological networks

3.5   Conclusions

The monitoring and evaluation instruments available to the Observatory on oncological networks provide information and data sources that, when integrated and made interoperable, help to identify the level of clinical, organizational, managerial and economic-financial performance of the single Regional oncological networks. This makes the intervention of the Observatory increasingly penetrating and targeted for the institutional aims it has been commissioned with.

The Observatory is, therefore, of fundamental importance, as it ensures the collection of data from the Regional oncological networks and the transmission of integrated data at regional and/or national level.

In conclusion, the Observatory on oncological networks is the necessary infrastructure that allows the progressive cultural growth of the system by promoting the exchange of expertise, knowledge and experience. As such, it should be regarded as having a strategic role in the overall enhancement of the quality of the National Healthcare Service.

Acknowledgments We would like to appreciate all professionals who collaborated to the drawing up of the document for the Agreement of April 17, 2019 between the Government, the Regions and the Autonomous Provinces of Trento and Bolzano: they are all listed at the end of that document.
Many thanks to Giacomo Giolo, Lisa Baldini, Maria Rita Cafulli and Stella Lanzi for editing and English translation.

References

1. Ministero della Salute. Decreto ministeriale 2 aprile 2015 n. 70, "Regolamento recante definizione degli standard qualitativi, strutturali, tecnologici e quantitativi relativi all'assistenza ospedaliera" [Ministry of Health. Ministerial Decree April 2, 2015, n. 70, "Regulation on the definition of quality, structural, technological and quantitative standards relating to hospital care"]. https://www.gazzettaufficiale.it/eli/id/2015/06/04/15G00084/sg.
2. Accordo, ai sensi del punto 8.1 dell'Allegato 1 al decreto ministeriale 2 aprile 2015, n. 70, sul documento "Linee guida per la revisione delle reti cliniche - Le reti tempo dipendenti". Conferenza Permanente per i Rapporti tra lo Stato, le Regioni e le Province Autonome di Trento e Bolzano, 24 gennaio 2018 [Agreement, pursuant to point 8.1 of Annex 1 to the ministerial decree, April 2, 2015, n. 70, on the document "Guidelines for the review of clinical networks - Time dependent networks". Permanent Conference for Relations between the State, the Regions and the Autonomous Provinces of Trento and Bolzano, January 24, 2018]. http://archivio.statoregioni.it/Documenti/DOC_063280_P.%209%20%20CSR%20Atto%20 Rep.%2014%20%2024gen2018.pdf.
3. Intesa, ai sensi dell'articolo 8, comma 6, della legge 5 giugno 2003, n. 131, tra il Governo, le Regioni e le Province autonome di Trento e Bolzano concernente il "Documento tecnico di indirizzo per ridurre il burden del cancro - Anni 2014–2016". 30 ottobre 2014 [Agreement, pursuant to article 8, paragraph 6, of the law of June 5, 2003, n. 131, between the Government, the Regions and the Autonomous Provinces of Trento and Bolzano concerning the "Technical Guidance Document to reduce the burden of cancer—Years 2014–2016". October 30, 2014]. http://www.salute.gov.it/imgs/C_17_pubblicazioni_2324_allegato.pdf.

4. Accordo, ai sensi dell'articolo 4, del decreto legislativo 28 agosto 1997, n. 281, tra il Governo, le Regioni e le Province autonome di Trento e di Bolzano sul documento recante "Revisione delle Linee Guida organizzative e delle raccomandazioni per la Rete Oncologica che integra l'attività ospedaliera per acuti e post acuti con l'attività territoriale". 17 Aprile 2019 [Agreement, pursuant to Article 4, of legislative decree August 28, 1997, n. 281, between the Government, the Regions and the Autonomous Provinces of Trento and Bolzano on the document "Revision of the Organizational Guidelines and recommendations for the Oncology Network which integrates hospital activities for acute and post-acute patients with territorial activity". April 17, 2019]. http://www.statoregioni.it/media/1614/p-2-csr-atti-rep-n-59-17apr2019.pdf.
5. Agenzia Nazionale per i Servizi Sanitari Regionali. Deliberazione n. 455 del 2 agosto 2019. Istituzione dell'Osservatorio per il monitoraggio e la valutazione delle reti oncologiche. [National Agency for Regional Health Services. Resolution n. 455 of August 2, 2019 Establishment of the Observatory for monitoring and evaluation of regional cancer networks]. https://www.agenas.gov.it/images/agenas/RETI/DELIBERA_455-2019.pdf.

Volume-Outcome Relationship in Esophageal Surgery

4

Jacopo Weindelmayer, Luca Alberti,
Carlo Alberto De Pasqual, and Giovanni de Manzoni

4.1   Introduction

Esophageal cancer is the seventh most common cause of cancer-related death [1]. The two main histological subtypes are adenocarcinoma and squamous cell carcinoma, which account for 98% of all esophageal tumors and have different risk factors and incidence rates. Gastroesophageal reflux disease is the main risk factor for adenocarcinoma, and Barrett's esophagus is a well-known precursor of esophageal adenocarcinoma. Obesity also seems to be associated with a higher risk of esophageal adenocarcinoma. Tobacco smoking and alcohol abuse are the main risk factors for squamous cell carcinoma. The different patterns of disease described worldwide are the consequence of these different risk factors. In the West, the incidence of distal esophageal/gastroesophageal junction adenocarcinoma has been steadily increasing over the last 50 years [2]. As a result, adenocarcinoma is now the most frequent subtype observed in North America, Europe and Australia. By contrast, the reduction in smoking habit and alcohol abuse in these countries has led to a decrease in the incidence of squamous cell carcinoma. This subtype remains the most frequently diagnosed in Central and South East Asia [3]. Both histotypes have a poor prognosis, with an overall 5-year survival rate ranging from 20 to 30% [4].

Surgery is the mainstay of curative treatment for esophageal cancer, either alone or as a part of a multimodal approach. However, despite the improvements in surgical techniques and perioperative management, the morbidity and mortality rates remain considerable and esophagectomy is considered a high-risk procedure also in high-volume centers [5]. In 1979 Luft et al. [6] published the first report about the

J. Weindelmayer · L. Alberti · C. A. De Pasqual · G. de Manzoni (✉)
Division of General and Upper Gastrointestinal Surgery, Department of Surgery,
Dentistry, Pediatrics and Gynecology, University of Verona, Verona, Italy
e-mail: j.weindelmayer@gmail.com; lucaalberti90@gmail.com;
carlodepasqual@gmail.com; giovanni.demanzoni@univr.it

© Springer Nature Switzerland AG 2021   25
M. Montorsi (ed.), *Volume-Outcome Relationship in Oncological Surgery*,
Updates in Surgery, https://doi.org/10.1007/978-3-030-51806-6_4

relationship between surgical volume and the reduction of hospital mortality. Since then, several studies have demonstrated the role of both hospital and surgeon volume in improving short-term postoperative outcomes [7, 8].

One of the first studies to suggest a similar association after esophagectomy was published by Birkmeyer et al. in 2002 [9]. Even though the authors did not identify any specific volume thresholds to optimize outcomes, they stated that a high volume decreases the odds of mortality. They demonstrated, in a subsequent paper, a similar volume-outcome relationship when considering the annual number of esophagectomies performed by a single surgeon [10].

Several factors should be taken into account to explain these advantages. Experience of the surgeon and of all the care providers involved in the surgery and perioperative management plays an important role but it is not the sole determinant of outcome. The presence of a multidisciplinary board to ensure appropriate clinical staging, the indication for adjuvant/neoadjuvant treatment as well as the surgical indication are key factors in optimizing patient management [11].

Despite this well-known evidence, the centralization of esophageal surgery has been implemented in only a few healthcare systems. For instance, the British National Health System (NHS) began a policy of mandatory centralization of esophagectomy in 2003. The number of centers performing this surgical procedure was reduced from 113 centers to only 43 in 10 years, and the 90-day mortality decreased from 11.3% in 2003 to 4.6% in 2014. However, in such a long period, many other factors—unrelated to the volume-outcome relationship—may have contributed to this reduction [12].

Other healthcare systems, as in the US, still do not have a federal centralization policy. In these countries several initiatives to encourage centralization have been carried out by private associations, such as the Leapfrog Group. In their 2020 report on hospital performances, they set the minimum annual volume of esophagectomies to be 20 for the hospital and 7 for the surgeon to achieve their quality standard [13]. A similar effort towards regionalization is the "Take the Volume Pledge", publicly announced by three major academic teaching hospitals in 2015. This pledge challenged the other large health systems to join them in restricting the performance of 10 surgical procedures—including gastrointestinal, cardiovascular, and joint-replacement surgeries—to hospitals and surgeons who perform more than a minimum number.

In these healthcare systems some observers report a peculiar process of "spontaneous centralization", which consists of a passive migration of patients towards high-volume centers.

For instance, in 2015 Munasinghe et al. [14] published a comparison of esophagectomy outcomes between England and the US: over the period 2005–2010 they reported a reduction in the number of hospitals performing esophagectomies of 27% in England (a country with a mandatory centralization policy) and 24% in US, where there was no government-endorsed policy.

In 2018, Schlottmann et al. [15] confirmed this trend, describing a significant increase in the percentage of esophagectomies performed in high-volume centers in the US, from 29.2% in 2000 to 68.5% in 2011 ($p < 0.0001$). In association with these findings, they reported a decrease in overall mortality rates from 10% in 2000 to 3.5% in 2011.

A possible limitation of the process of spontaneous migration of patients is related to socioeconomic aspects. Some authors in fact revealed that the patients who move towards high-volume centers are more likely to be younger [16], to be white, to have a private insurance and to have a lower Charlson comorbidity score [17].

Finally, an interesting aspect of regionalization concerns healthcare costs [18]. Several studies reported that length of hospital stay [19] and postoperative complications are the strongest drivers of cost after esophagectomy [20]. It seems to be intuitive that in centers with enhanced recovery protocols and low morbidity-mortality the costs of esophagectomy may decrease, with possible significant cost savings [19, 21].

In conclusion, a consensus about what should be considered a high-volume hospital and minimum volume standards has not yet been achieved, and the definitions vary by country and region. As previously seen, the American Leapfrog group fixed the standard at 20 esophagectomies, as in the Netherlands. In Great Britain a high-volume center is defined at 60 gastroesophageal cancer resections per year. In Italy, as discussed below, no formal policy is available and the efforts to define a cut-off value are restricted to regional regulations.

4.2   Short-Term Outcomes (Surgical Outcomes)

Esophagectomy is one of the most demanding surgical procedures, burdened by high morbidity and mortality rates even in high-volume centers. The Esophageal Complications Consensus Group (ECCG) published a study on 2704 resections performed in 24 high-volume esophageal surgical centers in 14 countries. The authors reported a 30-day and 90-day mortality of 2.4% and 4.5%, respectively. The overall incidence of complications was 59%. Severe complications (Clavien-Dindo complications ≥IIIb) occurred in 17.2% of patients [5].

4.2.1   Postoperative Mortality

In recent years several studies have focused on the relationship between hospital volume and postoperative mortality (Table 4.1).

In an impressive series of more than 23,000 esophagectomies [22], Fuchs et al. reported that the overall mortality of patients who underwent esophageal surgery in low-volume centers (defined as centers that performed less than 6 cases/year) was more than twice the mortality of those who were treated in high-volume hospitals (>20 esophagectomies/year) (11.4% in low-volume centers vs. 4.0% in high-volume centers; $p < 0.05$).

In a quantitative meta-analysis of volume-outcome following esophagectomy, comprising 27,843 operations in low- and high-volume surgical units [23] Markar

Table 4.1 Studies on the relationship between center or surgeon volume and postoperative mortality in esophagectomy

Authors	Country	N. of patients	Group volume	Threshold	Mortality (%)	p-value
Sclhottmann, 2018 [15]	USA	5235	Low-volume centers High-volume centers	<5 >20	10.2 3.9	p < 0.0001
Fuchs, 2016 [22]	USA	23,751	Low-volume centers High-volume centers	<6 >20	11.4 4.01	p < 0.05
Markar, 2012 [23]	European Union	27,843	Low-volume centers High-volume centers	4–10 9–80	7.69 2.29	p < 0.0001
Wouters, 2009 [33]	The Netherlands	903	Low-volume centers High-volume centers	<7	13 5	p < 0.001
Dikken, 2015 [34]	European Union	10,854	Low-volume centers High-volume centers	<11 >41	7.2 4.3	p < 0.001
Fumagalli, 2013 [35] [a]	Italy	2801	Low-volume centers High-volume centers	<50 >150	5.7 1.7	p < 0.001
Modrall, 2018 [36]	USA	26,795	Low-volume surgeon High-volume surgeon	<5 >5	7.7 3.8	p < 0.001

[a]Esophagectomy and gastrectomy

et al. demonstrated a significant increase in 30-day (2.09% vs. 0.73%; $p < 0.0001$) and in-hospital mortality (8.48% vs. 2.82%; $p < 0.0001$) in low-volume centers. However, the thresholds considered for defining "low-volume centers" in the studies analyzed were very low, ranging from 4 to 10 operations/year.

Confirmation of the improved outcomes related to centralization comes from a retrospective study comparing 7433 esophagectomies performed in 66 English hospitals (a health system with a centralization policy) and 5858 esophagectomies in 775 US hospitals [14] (no centralization policy for esophageal surgery). A first analysis revealed that the in-hospital mortality was higher in the US than in England

(5.5% vs. 4.2%; $p = 0.001$). However, when comparing US and UK high-volume institutions, the US mortality dropped to 60% of that observed in England. The US authors of this paper strongly recommend supporting the continued centralization of high-risk cancer procedures in an effort to reduce perioperative mortality.

4.2.2 Postoperative Morbidity

Until recently there was no standardized classification for complications after esophagectomy. Only in 2015 did an international consensus group, involving the most important esophageal centers from all around the world, publish a standardized classification of complications after esophagectomy [24]. As a consequence, it is difficult to compare the morbidity rates reported in studies published before 2015. Moreover, most of the studies still refer to hospital mortality as the sole outcome measure.

An index that may reflect surgical outcomes is the length of hospital stay. In 2017, Giwa et al. conducted a meta-analysis with 75,383 patients from the USA, UK, Canada, the Netherlands, southern Australia, and Japan showing a 4% decrease in the risk of a length of stay ≥14 days for every additional five esophagectomy cases at a hospital per year [25].

Two conclusions can be drawn: firstly, that surgeons performing a high number of esophagectomies are more confident in discharging uncomplicated patients early; secondly, that the experience of the team plays a crucial role in promptly recognizing and treating postoperative complications, leading to a shorter stay and a better clinical outcome.

Even though a higher rate of postoperative complications (in particular respiratory failure and bleeding) has been described in low-volume centers [15], some authors suggested that the main determinant of the poorer results is not the higher incidence of complications itself but, rather, the inability to rescue patients who suffer from a major complication. Ghaferi et al. reported a 3.2 times greater odds of failure to rescue after esophagectomy in very low-volume hospitals (<4 per year) compared to very high-volume hospitals (>15 per year) [26]. Nimptsch et al. reported in 2018 a different ability to rescue patients from complications in high-/low-volume centers. In-hospital mortality of complicated patients was 20% in very low-volume centers (<2 esophagectomies per year) compared with 12.3% in high-volume centers (>62 esophagectomies per year) [27].

The management of complications for esophageal surgery involves several care processes (intraoperative anesthesia support, postoperative critical care management, enhanced recovery protocols, endoscopy [4], interventional radiology) which are crucial to treat postoperative complications properly [28] and which may have more impact on clinical outcomes than individual surgeon experience.

Funk et al. [29] identified five key characteristics (high nurse ratios, lung transplantation services, complex medical oncology services, bariatric surgery services and positron emission tomography scanners) with a meaningful impact on determining postoperative outcomes. In their paper they stated that at least 3 out of 5 items need to be present to reach a significantly lower mortality rate (12.5% vs. 5.0%; $p = 0.042$).

4.3   Long-Term Outcomes (Oncological Outcomes)

The long-term outcomes of patients with esophageal cancer depend on several factors. Among them, a main role is played by appropriate oncological assessment and surgical expertise.

A multidisciplinary evaluation is mandatory to define a tailored diagnostic-therapeutic pathway. A multimodal strategy, combining chemotherapy, radiotherapy and surgery, in either a neoadjuvant or adjuvant setting, has been associated with improved long-term outcomes. A stable multidisciplinary board dedicated to the evaluation of upper gastrointestinal tumors is more frequently present in facilities that treat a high number of patients.

In esophageal malignancies, it is well recognized that both neoadjuvant chemotherapy and chemo-radiotherapy improve overall and disease-free survival.

A first demonstration of the relationship between high-volume hospital and oncological treatment was provided by a retrospective study [30] of 5016 patients from 305 cancer care hospitals in Japan. The analysis revealed that patients were subjected to neoadjuvant therapy less frequently in the low-volume hospitals than in the high-volume centers (very high, 42.1%; high, 37.5%; low, 30.7%; and very low, 26.4%).

Similarly, Chapman et al. [31] described that, in the US, patients treated in hospitals performing 10 or more esophagectomies per year were more likely to receive neoadjuvant therapy than patients cared for in hospitals performing less than 10 esophagectomies per year ($p < 0.001$). Moreover, this study demonstrated a substantial survival advantage in patients undergoing treatment at facilities performing 20 or more esophagectomies per year, adjusting for patient and tumor-related characteristics.

An appropriate surgical resection is a key point in the treatment of esophageal neoplasms. The aims of the surgery are to achieve an R0 resection (microscopically margin-negative resection) and an adequate lymphadenectomy (at least 21 lymph nodes according to the TNM, 8th edition), and these parameters are often used as indicators of the quality of the surgery.

As for radicality of the resection, in the US a significantly higher rate of R1 resections has been reported in low-volume centers (<20 esophagectomies/year) compared to centers performing more than 20 esophagectomies (9.9% vs. 6.0%; $p < 0.001$) [32]. Moreover, the same authors reported that an adequate lymphadenectomy was more likely to be performed in high-volume centers. The rate of removal of at least 15 lymph nodes was 42.6% in high-volume centers compared to 18.5% of low-volume hospitals ($p < 0.001$). Speicher [17] confirmed these findings, demonstrating a significantly higher rate of harvested lymph nodes in high-volume centers (median number of lymph nodes was 17 in high-volume centers vs. 10 in low-volume centers; $p < 0.001$).

4.4   The Italian Perspective

According to the Italian National Agency for Regional Health Services (AGENAS), in 2017 a total of 843 esophagectomies were performed in 148 Italian hospitals. Of these, only 10 hospitals performed more than 20 esophagectomies per year and most of them were located in northern Italy, and specifically in two Italian Regions: Veneto and Lombardy. Nonetheless, esophagectomy continues to be performed all around the country, partly due to the lack of a formal centralization policy. Consequently, a minimum volume standard for esophagectomies in Italy is not available and attempts for its definition come from single initiatives. One of these is represented by a group of expert surgeons in gastroesophageal resection [4] who identified the minimum cut-off for a high-volume center at 20 esophagectomies/year. Moreover, they added other structural and organizational requirements, aiming to define the minimal quality standards needed to obtain accreditation to perform esophageal surgery.

As a structural requirement the hospital must be able to offer:

- an endoscopy unit able to perform operative endoscopy and endoscopic ultrasound;
- a radiology unit;
- a pathology unit;
- an intensive care unit;
- an oncology unit;
- a radiotherapy unit;
- a physiotherapy unit;
- operating rooms equipped for minimally invasive procedures.

The organizational requirement regards the diagnostic-therapeutic pathway. The presence of a dedicated multidisciplinary board (including a surgeon, oncologist, radiologist, endoscopist, radiotherapist and pathologist) is mandatory. The board is meant to discuss every case at each step of the diagnostic-therapeutic process: at diagnosis, after neoadjuvant treatment, after surgery and during the follow-up, if needed.

The development and application of a perioperative multidisciplinary enhanced recovery program is recommended, including evaluation for respiratory physiotherapy and nutritional assessment.

Other concrete efforts to define a minimum volume standard include diagnostic, therapeutic and care pathways (PDTA, percorsi diagnostico-terapeutici assistenziali), confined to the regional context. An esophageal cancer PDTA is available in the Veneto and Piedmont Regions. For instance, the Veneto PDTA defines ten benchmarks as performance indicators for surgical-oncological centers (Table 4.2).

This proposal is a valid attempt to define a proper clinical pathway. However, such a complex process cannot be left to a single regional initiative. A strong policy driven by the national health system and supported by the scientific community

Table 4.2 Benchmarks as performance indicators (PDTA) for esophageal cancer in surgical-oncological centers of the Veneto Region, Italy

Indicators	Benchmark	Performance
Surgical volume	>20 procedures/ year	Surgical outcome
Discussion in multidisciplinary team	>90% of patients	Appropriate oncological assessment
R0 resection rate	>80%	Surgical outcome
Minimum nodes harvested	15 nodes	Surgical outcome
Tumor regression grade exams	100%	Appropriate diagnostic assessment
Starting of neoadjuvant treatment within 6 weeks from diagnosis	100%	Appropriate treatment
90-day mortality rate	<5%	Surgical outcome
30-day mortality or in hospital mortality rate	<3%	Surgical outcome
Terminal patient with a guaranteed palliative care path	>70%	Appropriate pathways of care
Patients with a chemotherapy treatment received 30 days before death	<10%	Appropriate pathways of care

PDTA Diagnostic, therapeutic and care pathways (Percorsi diagnostico terapeutici assistenziali)

must be established in order to share common healthcare provision and deliver the best healthcare for oncological patients.

References

1. Global Burden of Disease Cancer Collaboration, Fitzmaurice C, Akinyemiju TF, Al Lami FH, et al. Global, regional, and national cancer incidence, mortality, years of life lost, years lived with disability, and disability-adjusted life-years for 29 cancer groups, 1990 to 2016: a systematic analysis for the global burden of disease study. JAMA Oncol. 2018;4(11):1553–68.
2. Bray F, Ferlay J, Soerjomataram I, et al. Global cancer statistics 2018: GLOBOCAN estimates of incidence and mortality worldwide for 36 cancers in 185 countries. CA Cancer J Clin. 2018;68(6):394–424.
3. Thrift A. The epidemic of esophageal carcinoma: where are we now? Cancer Epidemiol. 2016;41:88–95.
4. Parise P, Elmore U, Fumagalli U, et al. Esophageal surgery in Italy. Criteria to identify the hospital units and the tertiary referral centers entitled to perform it. Updat Surg. 2016;68(2):129–33.
5. Low DE, Kuppusamy MK, Alderson D, et al. Benchmarking complications associated with esophagectomy. Ann Surg. 2019;269(2):291–8.
6. Luft HS, Bunker JP, Enthoven AC. Should operations be regionalized? The empirical relation between surgical volume and mortality. N Engl J Med. 1979;301(25):1364–9.
7. Urbach DR. Pledging to eliminate low volume surgery. N Engl J Med. 2015;373(15):1388–90.
8. Begg CB, Cramer LD, Hoskins WJ, Brennan MF. Impact of hospital volume on operative mortality in the United States. JAMA. 1998;280(20):1747–51.
9. Birkmeyer JD, Siewers AE, Finlayson EV, et al. Hospital volume and surgical mortality in the United States. N Engl J Med. 2002;346(15):1128–37.
10. Birkmeyer JD, Stukel TA, Siewers AE, et al. Surgeon volume and operative mortality in the United States. N Engl J Med. 2003;349:2117–27.
11. Glatz T, Hopper J. Is there a rationale for structural quality assurance in esophageal surgery? Visc Med. 2017;33(2):135–9.

12. Varagunam M, Hardwick R, Riley S, et al. Changes in volume, clinical practice and outcome after reorganisation of oesophago-gastric cancer care in England: a longitudinal observational study. Eur J Surg Oncol. 2018;44(4):524–31.
13. The Leapfrog Group. Leapfrog Hospital Survey—Factsheet: Inpatient Surgery (revision: 4 January 2020). https://www.leapfroggroup.org/sites/default/files/Files/2020%20Surgical%20 Volume-Appropriateness%20Fact%20Sheet.pdf. Accessed 30 Apr 2020.
14. Munasinghe A, Markar SR, Mamidanna R, et al. Is it time to centralize high-risk cancer care in the United States? Comparison of outcomes of esophagectomy between England and the United States. Ann Surg. 2015;262(1):79–85.
15. Schlottmann F, Strassle P, Charles AG, et al. Esophageal cancer surgery: spontaneous centralization in the US contributed to reduce mortality without causing health disparities. Ann Surg Oncol. 2018;25(6):1580–7.
16. Song Y, Tieniber A, Roses R. National trends in centralization and perioperative outcomes of complex operations for cancer. Surgery. 2019;166(5):800–11.
17. Speicher PJ, Englum BR, Ganapathi AM, et al. Traveling to a high-volume center is associated with improved survival for patients with esophageal surgery. Ann Surg. 2017;265(4):743–9.
18. Clark JM, Boffa D, Meguid RA, et al. Regionalization of esophagectomy: where are we now? J Thorac Dis. 2019;11(Suppl 12):S1633–42.
19. Weindelmayer J, Verlato G, Alberti L, et al. Enhanced recovery protocol in esophagectomy, is it really worth it? A cost analysis related to team experience and protocol compliance. Dis Esophagus. 2019;32(8):doy114. https://doi.org/10.1093/dote/doy114.
20. Fischer C, Lingsma H, Klazinga N, et al. Volume-outcome revisited: the effect of hospital and surgeon volumes on multiple outcome measures in oesophago-gastric cancer surgery. PLoS One. 2017;12(10):e0183955. https://doi.org/10.1371/journal.pone.0183955.
21. Kennedy GT, Ukert BD, Predina JD, et al. Implications of hospital volume on costs following esophagectomy in the United States. J Gastrointest Surg. 2018;22(11):1845–51.
22. Fuchs H, Harnsberger C, Broderick RC, et al. Mortality after esophagectomy is heavily impacted by center volume: retrospective analysis of the Nationwide Inpatient Sample. Surg Endosc. 2016;3(6):2491–7.
23. Markar S, Karthikesalingam A, Thrumurthy S, Low DE. Volume-outcome relationship in surgery for esophageal malignancy: systematic review and meta-analysis 2000–2011. J Gastrointest Surg. 2012;16(5):1055–63.
24. Low D, Alderson D, Cecconello I, et al. International consensus on standardization of data collection for complications associated with esophagectomy: Esophagectomy Complications Consensus Group (ECCG). Ann Surg. 2015;262(2):286–94.
25. Giwa F, Salami A, Abioye AI. Hospital esophagectomy volume and postoperative length of stay: a systematic review and meta-analysis. Am J Surg. 2018;215(1):155–62.
26. Ghaferi AA, Birkmeyer JD, Dimick JB. Hospital volume and failure to rescue with high risk surgery. Med Care. 2011;49(12):1076–81.
27. Nimptsch U, Haist T, Krautz C, et al. Hospital volume, in-hospital mortality, and failure to rescue in esophageal surgery. Dtsch Arztebl Int. 2018;115(47):793–800.
28. Tol JA, van Gulik TM, Busch OR, Gouma DJ. Centralization of highly complex low volume procedures in upper gastrointestinal surgery. A summary of systematic reviews and meta-analysis. Dig Surg. 2012;29(5):374–83.
29. Funk LM, Gawande AA, Semel ME, et al. Esophagectomy outcomes at low-volume hospitals: the association between systems characteristics and mortality. Ann Surg. 2011;253(5):912–7.
30. Tsukada Y, Higashi T, Shimada H, et al. The use of neoadjuvant therapy for resectable locally advanced thoracic esophageal squamous cell carcinoma in an analysis of 5016 patients from 305 designated cancer care hospitals in Japan. Int J Clin Oncol. 2018;23(1):81–91.
31. Chapman B, Weyant M, Hilton S, et al. Analysis of the National Cancer Database esophageal squamous cell carcinoma in the United States. Ann Thorac Surg. 2019;108(5):1535–42.
32. Samson P, Puri V, Broderick S, et al. Adhering to quality measures in esophagectomy is associated with improved survival in all stages of esophageal cancer. Ann Thorac Surg. 2017;103(4):1101–8.

33. Wouters MW, Krijnen P, Le Cessie S, et al. Volume- or outcome-based referral to improve quality of care for esophageal cancer surgery in The Netherlands. J Surg Oncol. 2009;99:481–7.
34. Dikken JL, van Sandick JW, Allum WH, et al. Differences in outcomes of oesophageal and gastric cancer surgery across Europe. Br J Surg. 2015;100(1):83–94.
35. Fumagalli U, Bersani M, Russo A, et al. Volume and outcomes after esophageal cancer surgery: the experience of the Region of Lombardy—Italy. Updat Surg. 2013;65(4):271–5.
36. Modrall J, Minter R, Minhajuddin A. The surgeon volume-outcome relationship: not yet ready for policy. Ann Surg. 2018;267(5):863–7.

Volume-Outcome Relationship in Hepatobiliary Surgery

5

Matteo Donadon, Eloisa Franchi, and Guido Torzilli

5.1 Introduction

The positive relationship between volume and outcome in hepatobiliary surgery has been demonstrated for many years. As for other complex surgical procedures, both improved short- and long-term outcomes have been associated with a higher volume of procedures [1–15]. However, whether the centralization of complex hepatobiliary procedures makes full sense because it should be associated with higher quality of care, as reported in the literature, precise criteria on what to centralize, where to centralize, and who should be entitled to perform complex procedures are all aspects that remain to be elucidated. Indeed, despite the generalized consensus on centralization in hepatobiliary surgery, the subject is very complex because many determinants are involved in the centralization process, some of which cannot be easily controlled. In the context of different health systems worldwide, such as national health systems and private insurances, there are different stakeholders—politicians, patients, surgeons, institutions and medical associations—that do not always have the same needs.

Starting from the review of the literature on centralization in hepatobiliary surgery, this chapter will propose some guidelines that, when not data-driven due to low evidence levels in the literature, will be based on good clinical practice.

M. Donadon · G. Torzilli (✉)

Department of Biomedical Sciences, Humanitas University, Pieve Emanuele, Milan, Italy
Department of Hepatobiliary and General Surgery, Humanitas Clinical and Research Center IRCCS, Rozzano, Milan, Italy
e-mail: matteo.donadon@hunimed.eu; guido.torzilli@hunimed.eu

E. Franchi
Department of Hepatobiliary and General Surgery, Humanitas Clinical and Research Center IRCCS, Rozzano, Milan, Italy
e-mail: eloisa.franchi@humanitas.it

© Springer Nature Switzerland AG 2021

35

M. Montorsi (ed.), *Volume-Outcome Relationship in Oncological Surgery*,
Updates in Surgery, https://doi.org/10.1007/978-3-030-51806-6_5

5.2   Review of the Literature

A review of the literature regarding the relationship between outcome and volume in hepatobiliary surgery is detailed in Table 5.1. Considering the rapid evolution of liver surgery, we have included articles published in the last 20 years in English. Moreover, we have included only those articles that have distinguish hepatobiliary surgery from pancreatic surgery, which are usually considered together [14–44].

As detailed, almost all the included articles supported a positive relationship between hospital volume and outcome indicating the validity of the union high-volume and high-quality. In particular, Dimick et al. [19] analyzed more than 2000

Table 5.1 Review of the literature on the relationship between outcome and volume in hepatobiliary surgery

Author	N. of patients	Importance of center volume	Importance of surgeon volume
Begg et al. 1998 [17]	801	+	n/a
Choti et al. 1998 [16]	606	+	n/a
Glasgow et al. 1999 [20]	507	+	+
Gordon et al. 1999 [18]	293	+	+
Dimick et al. 2003 [19]	2097	+	+
Imamura et al. 2003 [21]	1056	+	+
Fong et al. 2005 [22]	3734	+	n/a
Hollenbeck et al. 2007 [23]	3630	+	n/a
Eppsteiner et al. 2008 [25]	2949	−	+
McKay et al. 2008 [24]	1107	+	+
Nathan et al. 2009 [27]	6871	+	−
Stella 2009 [26]	n/a	−	n/a
Chamberlain et al. 2011 [28]	84	−	+
Giuliante et al. 2012 [29]	588	+	n/a
Yasunaga et al. 2012 [30]	18,046	+	n/a
Viganò et al. 2013 [31]	106	+	n/a
Goetze et al. 2014 [33] [a]	487	+	n/a
Ravaioli et al. 2014 [32]	621	−	+
Schneider et al. 2014 [34]	3695	+	+
Spolverato et al. 2014 [14]	9874	+	n/a
Chang et al. 2014 [44]	13,159	+	+
Aldrighetti et al. 2015 [35] [b]	1497	+	n/a
Ejaz et al. 2015 [36]	9466	n/a	+
Buettner et al. 2016 [15]	5075	+	+
Gani et al. 2016 [37]	27,813	+	n/a
Botea et al. 2017 [39]	3016	+	+
Chapman et al. 2017 [38]	12,757	+	+
Idrees et al. 2018 [40]	96,107	+	n/a
Chen et al. 2019 [43]	4902	+	n/a
Filmann et al. 2019 [41]	110,332	+	+
Bouras et al. 2020 [42] [c]	46	−	n/a

n/a not available
[a]Focus on gallbladder cancer
[b]Focus on learning curve rather than hospital volume
[c]Focus on laparoscopic liver surgery

hepatectomies performed in North America and found that those institutions that performed more than 20 resections per year had significantly lower mortality rates (6.3% vs. 15.5%). In 2009 a systematic review and in 2012 a meta-analysis confirmed a reduced mortality risk after liver surgery in high-volume centers [45, 46]. Few of these articles, investigated whether this relationship was mainly based on hospital or organization factors rather than on surgeon factors. In general, the positive relationship was evident for both hospital and surgeon volumes. Even though this is reasonable, there are confounding factors that are difficult to separate. In this sense, it is important to note that is difficult to distinguish when high-quality care in complex surgery is the consequence of the reaching of the plateau of a learning curve or when is the consequence of a standard volume that is a minimum number of procedures per year.

Besides, it is important to note that good outcomes in hepatobiliary surgery are also related to the quality of other hospital services, such as the anesthesiology service and the intensive care unit, which similarly to the surgeons have to reach the plateau of their learning curves. In this sense, further studies should be conducted to better characterize these two phenomena (i.e., learning curve vs. minimum standard volume). Nathan et al. [27] reported that the surgeon volume was not associated with in-hospital mortality, while Chang et al. [44] reported that the combined effects of hospital and surgeon volume strongly influenced short-term survival after hepatic resection. In this latter study, the prognosis was adjusted for several different factors such as indication for surgery, quality of the underlying chronic liver disease, and socio-economic status that were found to be important to be recorded and analyzed to strengthen the relationship between perioperative outcome and surgeon and/or hospital volume. Chang et al. [44] also found that the combination high-volume surgeons in high-volume hospitals was associated with higher quality results, while the combination high-volume surgeons in low-volume hospitals was not. Notably, in this study high-volume hospitals were those institutions performing more than 245 cases per year, while high-volume surgeons were those surgeons performing more than 59 cases per year. Notwithstanding these published studies, the definition of "high-volume center" remains to be elucidated. There is no established cut-off number of liver resections to be performed per year [47].

5.3 Critical Issues Limiting the Centralization of Hepatobiliary Surgery

The goal of centralization of hepatobiliary surgery is to provide optimal care to patients affected by hepatobiliary diseases within a given geographical area. This centralization passes through a complex process of assessment, development of dedicated policies, ongoing assurance and support from national government agencies, which should have the competence and authority to promote high-quality care, good uses of technical and technological tools, good allocation of human resources, and at the same time monitor, minimize and control the probability of unfortunate events. This process should be provided along a space-time continuum that should warrant quality in all phases of the care of patients affected by hepatobiliary diseases.

These critical issues are particularly important in liver surgery for several reasons.

- *First*: the definition of resectability is not standardized and wide variability is observed among expert surgeons [48].
- *Second*: the complexity of liver surgery is difficult to be classified because several different types of resections requiring an extremely wide range of expertise can be performed. The standard distinction between major and minor hepatectomies is inadequate in the current era of modern liver surgery [49]. Indeed, there are different technical solutions allowing parenchymal-sparing hepatectomies, much more complex than standard major hepatectomies, that remain in the shadow of the definition of minor hepatectomy. Yet high-quality centers should not be considered those centers performing a high proportion of major hepatectomies. In this sense, a new classification for minor hepatectomy that might help in better reporting minor but complex resections has been recently proposed [50].
- *Third*: postoperative morbidity and mortality rates have a limited validity in assessing quality. Centers selecting only patients requiring small limited resections may have lower morbidity rates in comparison with centers routinely selecting patients requiring complex resections.
- *Fourth*: realistic cut-offs of mortality and morbidity rates after hepatectomy as a benchmark of quality should be defined to avoid the risk of denying care to those patients with higher complexity due to tumoral presentation or advanced age or because of severe comorbidities. Apart from the specificity of their indications for surgery, which needs to be addressed by the local multidisciplinary teams, risk-adjusted metrics to compare outcomes among institutions are mandatory. Otherwise the risk of unfair comparisons will remain. In this sense, a benchmarking process has been started by merging the comprehensive complications risk [51], liver failure occurrence, and morbidity and mortality classified according to the Clavien-Dindo classification [52]. Last but not least, as recently pointed out by Aloia et al. [53] there are some downsides to the strategy of aiming at zero mortality rates after surgery, such as the performance of innovative operations, which at least at the beginning are not compatible with perfection that might be strongly limited in the context of no-mortality.

Therefore, the centralization process in hepatobiliary surgery should pass through the development and adoption of a new and modern common language for indications, resectability, resection terminology, and good quality indicators.

5.4 Minimum Hospital Requirements in Hepatobiliary Surgery

To date, there are no specific published criteria that a given hospital should have to be able to perform hepatobiliary surgery. Most of the authors addressing this topic have reported their personal experiences, which should nonetheless be taken into consideration while awaiting data from some new studies.

In 2016 Torzilli et al. [54] published a position paper on behalf of the Italian Society of Surgery that had the merit of fueling the debate and setting some reference standards.

In Italy the current legislation on hospital standards is detailed by law n. 70/2015, which divides hospitals into three levels (i.e., basic, level I, and level II). Accordingly, hepatobiliary surgery should be performed in level I hospitals at least or even better in level II hospitals, and the surgical team should be dedicated only to hepatobiliary and/or hepatobiliary and pancreatic procedures. This dedication should guarantee high-quality standards. Moreover, those high-quality hospitals in which hepatobiliary surgery might be performed should have the following departments:

1. Department of Medical Oncology;
2. Department of Diagnostic Radiology, which should have some interventional radiologists dedicated to hepatobiliary diseases;
3. Department of Hepatology and/or of Internal Medicine with some internists dedicated to hepatobiliary diseases;
4. Department of Digestive Endoscopy;
5. Intensive Care Unit;
6. Department of Pathology;
7. Department of Nuclear Medicine;
8. Department of Radiation Oncology.

Even stating that the above-mentioned departments should be present in any high-quality hospital certified for hepatobiliary surgery, there might be the case of a given hospital that lacking some of those departments. In such a case, strong operative networks between that hospital and another institution should be activated to cover any deficiency. Similarly, in such a case of a given department of hepatobiliary surgery that does not provide liver transplantation, another referral center in the same geographical area should be in the network to give consultation for liver transplantation. It should no longer be possible for a patient with complex hepatobiliary disease hospitalized in a given hospital not entitled to perform diagnosis and/or therapy for that specific disease not to be provided with the required care through networking in the same geographical area.

5.5   Multidisciplinary Team

Nowadays, it is mandatory to have a multidisciplinary teams (MDT) dedicated to patients affected by hepatobiliary diseases. MDT meetings provide the correct global assessment of the patient both for the diagnosis and for the therapy. Any MDT meeting should include at least one member from the previously listed hospital departments to ensure that all aspects of care are covered. Only physicians dedicated to liver diseases should take part in the MDT meeting, which should be scheduled based on caseload, but in general once a week. A written report of the MDT should be provided for each patient with the signature of all the members that have contributed to the discussion. It is important to note that proper functioning of the MDT meeting relies on the proper combination of scientific evidence and local experience in the diagnosis and care of a given hepatobiliary disease. A well-balanced and authoritative MDT in terms of specialties represented provides better patient management and thus better short- and long-term outcomes [55–57].

5.6   Hospital Volume Versus Surgeon Volume

Ideally, hospital volume and surgeon volume should match, while in the real world this is not always the case. In hepatobiliary surgery, the relative importance of hospital volume vs. surgeon volume is very important because both short- and long-term outcomes are dependent on hospital factors, such as the presence of an intensive care unit, and surgeon factors, such as operative technique. Nathan et al. [27] showed that the protective effect of hospital hepatic resection volume persisted after case-mix adjustment for competing risk factors, while that was not the case considering the surgeon hepatic resection volume. Indeed, high- and low-volume surgeons had comparable in-hospital mortality rates after hepatectomy [27]. There are also other factors inherent to the hospital organization which were not considered and may have biased Nathan et al.'s conclusions: i.e., an active MDT meeting discussing each patient as stated above, which was overlooked by them and by many other authors as well.

5.7   Learning Curve or Standard Volume?

Center volume, surgeon volume, and surgeon experience all appear to impact success rates in liver surgery. A better understanding of how these factors interact to influence outcomes could help to develop specific healthcare strategies for improving the quality of care in patients with hepatobiliary diseases.

As previously stated, it is difficult to distinguish whether good outcomes in hepatobiliary surgery are more dependent on the learning curve or a minimum standard volume. A possible strategy to overcome this infertile dualism might be the introduction of certification for hepatobiliary surgeons. Far from the idea of more bureaucracy, this strategy might include the analysis of training with emphasis on the schools of surgery and mentorships that a given surgeon might have received during his or her training in complex hepatobiliary surgery. As recently pointed out by others, this was found to be a good strategy in the field of pancreatic surgery and might work also in other fields of surgery [32, 58]. Besides, it might be a way to reinforce the importance of the schools of surgery which, independently from the Universities, are those called upon to train young surgeons.

5.8   Toward Certified Hepatobiliary Surgeons

A strategy to overcome the difficulty in decoding the dualism between hospital volume and surgeon volume might be the introduction of certification provided by a national board of specialists. Similarly to the American Board of Surgery, which is an independent, non-profit organization founded for the purpose of certifying surgeons who have met a defined standard of education, training and knowledge, national specialist boards might work to define the minimum standard of care in hepatobiliary surgery on an individual basis. These boards might analyze the applicant's training and operative experience as well as his/her professionalism and ethics. Upon successful completion of these analyses, the surgeon could be granted hepatobiliary surgery certification by the board. This certification could serve as a prerequisite for good practice in hepatobiliary surgery, which combined with the above minimum hospital requirements in hepatobiliary surgery, both as a single institution and as an established network of different institutions, would guarantee high-quality care – independently from the number of procedures. Notably once certified, the hepatobiliary surgeon would have to undergo a process of recertification (every 5–10 years) to demonstrate ongoing professionalism and commitment to continuing medical education in the field of hepatobiliary surgery.

5.9   Conclusions

In conclusion, volume and outcome data in hepatobiliary surgery suffer several intrinsic limitations. Published studies are mostly observational and retrospective. Besides, the centralization process requires preparatory and preliminary agreements among experts about the development and adoption of a new and modern common language for indications, resectability, terminology of resection, and good quality indicators. Without these agreements, hospital and surgeon volume act as proxy measures for technical and nontechnical skills. However, such centralization process remains very important to offer better care to patients undergoing complex hepatobiliary surgery.

References

1. Luft HS, Bunker JP, Enthoven AC. Should operations be regionalized? The empirical relation between surgical volume and mortality. N Engl J Med. 1979;301(25):1364–9.
2. Luft HS. The relation between surgical volume and mortality: an exploration of causal factors and alternative models. Med Care. 1980;18(9):940–59.
3. Gordon TA, Burleyson GP, Tielsch JM, Cameron JL. The effects of regionalization on cost and outcome for one general high-risk surgical procedure. Ann Surg. 1995;221(1):43–9.
4. Birkmeyer JD, Siewers AE, Finlayson EV, et al. Hospital volume and surgical mortality in the United States. N Engl J Med. 2002;346(15):1128–37.
5. Finlayson EV, Goodney PP, Birkmeyer JD. Hospital volume and operative mortality in cancer surgery: a national study. Arch Surg. 2003;138(7):721–5; discussion 726.
6. Birkmeyer JD, Stukel TA, Siewers AE, et al. Surgeon volume and operative mortality in the United States. N Engl J Med. 2003;349(22):2117–27.
7. Dimick JB, Pronovost PJ, Cowan JA Jr, Lipsett PA. Postoperative complication rates after hepatic resection in Maryland hospitals. Arch Surg. 2003;138(1):41–6.
8. Dimick JB, Wainess RM, Cowan JA, et al. National trends in the use and outcomes of hepatic resection. J Am Coll Surg. 2004;199(1):31–8.
9. Finks JF, Osborne NH, Birkmeyer JD. Trends in hospital volume and operative mortality for high-risk surgery. N Engl J Med. 2011;364(22):2128–37.

10. Liu JH, Zingmond DS, McGory ML, et al. Disparities in the utilization of high-volume hospitals for complex surgery. JAMA. 2006;296(16):1973–80.
11. Pearse RM, Moreno RP, Bauer P, et al. Mortality after surgery in Europe: a 7 day cohort study. Lancet. 2012;380(9847):1059–65.
12. Bauer H, Honselmann KC. Minimum volume standards in surgery—are we there yet? Visc Med. 2017;33(2):106–16.
13. Morche J, Mathes T, Pieper D. Relationship between surgeon volume and outcomes: a systematic review of systematic reviews. Syst Rev. 2016;5(1):204. https://doi.org/10.1186/s13643-016-0376-4.
14. Spolverato G, Ejaz A, Hyder O, et al. Failure to rescue as a source of variation in hospital mortality after hepatic surgery. Br J Surg. 2014;101(7):836–46.
15. Buettner S, Gani F, Amini N, et al. The relative effect of hospital and surgeon volume on failure to rescue among patients undergoing liver resection for cancer. Surgery. 2016;159(4):1004–12.
16. Choti MA, Bowman HM, Pitt HA, et al. Should hepatic resections be performed at high-volume referral centers? J Gastrointest Surg. 1998;2(1):11–20.
17. Begg CB, Cramer LD, Hoskins WJ, Brennan MF. Impact of hospital volume on operative mortality for major cancer surgery. JAMA. 1998;280(20):1747–51.
18. Gordon TA, Bowman HM, Bass EB, et al. Complex gastrointestinal surgery: impact of provider experience on clinical and economic outcomes. J Am Coll Surg. 1999;189(1):46–56.
19. Dimick JB, Cowan JA Jr, Knol JA, Upchurch GR Jr. Hepatic resection in the United States: indications, outcomes, and hospital procedural volumes from a nationally representative database. Arch Surg. 2003;138(2):185–91.
20. Glasgow RE, Showstack JA, Katz PP, et al. The relationship between hospital volume and outcomes of hepatic resection for hepatocellular carcinoma. Arch Surg. 1999;134(1):30–5.
21. Imamura H, Seyama Y, Kokudo N, et al. One thousand fifty-six hepatectomies without mortality in 8 years. Arch Surg. 2003;138(11):1198–206.
22. Fong Y, Gonen M, Rubin D, et al. Long-term survival is superior after resection for cancer in high-volume centers. Ann Surg. 2005;242(4):540–7.
23. Hollenbeck BK, Dunn RL, Miller DC, et al. Volume-based referral for cancer surgery: informing the debate. J Clin Oncol. 2007;25(1):91–6.
24. McKay A, You I, Bigam D, et al. Impact of surgeon training on outcomes after resective hepatic surgery. Ann Surg Oncol. 2008;15(5):1348–55.
25. Eppsteiner RW, Csikesz NG, Simons JP, et al. High volume and outcome after liver resection: surgeon or center? J Gastrointest Surg. 2008;12(10):1709–16.
26. Stella M. Safety and feasibility of liver resection at low-volume institutions. Surgery. 2009;145(5):575.
27. Nathan H, Cameron JL, Choti MA, et al. The volume-outcomes effect in hepato-pancreato-biliary surgery: hospital versus surgeon contributions and specificity of the relationship. J Am Coll Surg. 2009;208(4):528–38.
28. Chamberlain RS, Klaassen Z, Paragi PR. Complex hepatobiliary surgery in the community setting: is it safe and feasible? Am J Surg. 2011;202(3):273–80.
29. Giuliante F, Ardito F, Pinna AD, et al. Liver resection for hepatocellular carcinoma ≤3 cm: results of an Italian multicenter study on 588 patients. J Am Coll Surg. 2012;215(2):244–54.
30. Yasunaga H, Horiguchi H, Matsuda S, et al. Relationship between hospital volume and operative mortality for liver resection: data from the Japanese Diagnosis Procedure Combination database. Hepatol Res. 2012;42(11):1073–80.
31. Viganò L, Langella S, Ferrero A, Russolillo N, Sperti E, Capussotti L. Colorectal cancer with synchronous resectable liver metastases: monocentric management in a hepatobiliary referral center improves survival outcomes. Ann Surg Oncol. 2013;20(3):938–45.
32. Ravaioli M, Pinna AD, Francioni G, et al. A partnership model between high- and low-volume hospitals to improve results in hepatobiliary pancreatic surgery. Ann Surg. 2014;260(5):871–5; discussion 875–7.
33. Goetze TO, Paolucci V. Influence of high- and low-volume liver surgery in gallbladder carcinoma. World J Gastroenterol. 2014;20(48):18445–51.

34. Schneider EB, Ejaz A, Spolverato G, et al. Hospital volume and patient outcomes in hepato-pancreatico-biliary surgery: is assessing differences in mortality enough? J Gastrointest Surg. 2014;18(12):2105–15.
35. Aldrighetti L, Belli G, Boni L, et al. Italian experience in minimally invasive liver surgery: a national survey. Updat Surg. 2015;67(2):129–40.
36. Ejaz A, Spolverato G, Kim Y, et al. The impact of resident involvement on surgical outcomes among patients undergoing hepatic and pancreatic resections. Surgery. 2015;158(2):323–30.
37. Gani F, Pawlik TM. Assessing the costs associated with volume-based referral for hepatic surgery. J Gastrointest Surg. 2016;20(5):945–52.
38. Chapman BC, Paniccia A, Hosokawa PW, et al. Impact of facility type and surgical volume on 10-year survival in patients undergoing hepatic resection for hepatocellular carcinoma. J Am Coll Surg. 2017;224(3):362–72.
39. Botea F, Ionescu M, Braşoveanu V, et al. Liver resections in a high-volume center: from standard procedures to extreme surgery and ultrasound-guided resections. Chirurgia (Bucur). 2017;112(3):259–77.
40. Idrees JJ, Kimbrough CW, Rosinski BF, et al. The cost of failure: assessing the cost-effectiveness of rescuing patients from major complications after liver resection using the national inpatient sample. J Gastrointest Surg. 2018;22(10):1688–96.
41. Filmann N, Walter D, Schadde E, et al. Mortality after liver surgery in Germany. Br J Surg. 2019;106(11):1523–9.
42. Bouras AF, Liddo G, Marx-Deseure A, et al. Accessible laparoscopic liver resection performed in low volume centers: is it time for democratization? J Visc Surg. 2020;157(3):193–7. https://doi.org/10.1016/j.jviscsurg.2019.10.003.
43. Chen Q, Olsen G, Bagante F, et al. Procedure-specific volume and nurse-to-patient ratio: implications for failure to rescue patients following liver surgery. World J Surg. 2019;43(10):910–9.
44. Chang CM, Yin WY, Wei CK, et al. The combined effects of hospital and surgeon volume on short-term survival after hepatic resection in a population-based study. PLoS One. 2014;9(1):e86444. https://doi.org/10.1371/journal.pone.0086444.
45. Garcea G, Breukink SO, Marlow NE, et al. A systematic review of the impact of volume of hepatic surgery on patient outcome. Surgery. 2009;145(5):467–75.
46. Tol JA, van Gulik TM, Busch OR, Gouma DJ. Centralization of highly complex low-volume procedures in upper gastrointestinal surgery. A summary of systematic reviews and meta-analyses. Dig Surg. 2012;29(5):374–83.
47. Gruen RL, Pitt V, Green S, et al. The effect of provider case volume on cancer mortality: systematic review and meta-analysis. CA Cancer J Clin. 2009;59(3):192–211.
48. Folprecht G, Gruenberger T, Bechstein WO, et al. Tumour response and secondary resectability of colorectal liver metastases following neoadjuvant chemotherapy with cetuximab: the CELIM randomised phase 2 trial. Lancet Oncol. 2010;11(1):38–47.
49. Terminology Committee of the International Hepato-Pancreato-Biliary Association. The Brisbane 2000 terminology of liver anatomy and resections. HPB Surg. 2000;2(3):333–9.
50. Viganò L, Torzilli G, Troisi R, et al. Minor hepatectomies: focusing a blurred picture: analysis of the outcome of 4471 open resections in patients without cirrhosis. Ann Surg. 2019;270(5):842–51.
51. Slankamenac K, Graf R, Barkun J, et al. The comprehensive complication index: a novel continuous scale to measure surgical morbidity. Ann Surg. 2013;258(1):1–7.
52. Rössler F, Sapisochin G, Song G, et al. Defining benchmarks for major liver surgery: a multicenter analysis of 5202 living liver donors. Ann Surg. 2016;264(3):492–500.
53. Aloia TA. Should zero harm be our goal? Ann Surg. 2019;271(1):33–6.
54. Torzilli G, Viganò L, Giuliante F, Pinna AD. Liver surgery in Italy. Criteria to identify the hospital units and the tertiary referral centers entitled to perform it. Updat Surg. 2016;68(2):135–42.
55. Yopp AC, Mansour JC, Beg MS, et al. Establishment of a multidisciplinary hepatocellular carcinoma clinic is associated with improved clinical outcome. Ann Surg Oncol. 2014;21(4):1287–95.

56. Gashin L, Tapper E, Babalola A, et al. Determinants and outcomes of adherence to recommendations from a multidisciplinary tumour conference for hepatocellular carcinoma. HPB (Oxford). 2014;16(11):1009–15.
57. Viganò L, Pedicini V, Comito T, et al. Aggressive and multidisciplinary local approach to iterative recurrences of colorectal liver metastases. World J Surg. 2018;42(8):2651–9.
58. Capretti G, Balzano G, Gianotti L, et al. Management and outcomes of pancreatic resections performed in high-volume referral and low-volume community hospitals lead by surgeons who shared the same mentor: the importance of training. Dig Surg. 2018;35(1):42–8.

Volume-Outcome Relationship in Pancreatic Surgery

6

Gianpaolo Balzano, Claudio Bassi, Giulia Caraceni,
Massimo Falconi, Marco Montorsi, and Alessandro Zerbi

6.1 Introduction

Pancreatic surgery has been traditionally considered a high-risk surgery. Despite the improvement of surgical techniques and postoperative care, the morbidity and mortality rates are still high, ranging between 30–60% and 1–5%, respectively [1, 2]. During the last few decades, the centralization of pancreatic resections in high-volume hospitals has been the intervention that most has contributed to the drastic reduction of mortality. Therefore, an urgent need has emerged to identify which

G. Balzano · M. Falconi
Division of Pancreatic Surgery, Pancreas Translational and Clinical Research Center, San Raffaele Scientific Institute, Milan, Italy
e-mail: balzano.gianpaolo@hsr.it; falconi.massimo@hsr.it

C. Bassi
Department of General and Pancreatic Surgery, Pancreas Institute, University and Hospital Trust of Verona, G.B. Rossi Hospital, University of Verona, Verona, Italy
e-mail: claudio.bassi@univr.it

G. Caraceni
Pancreatic Surgery Unit, Humanitas Clinical and Research Center IRCCS, Rozzano, Milan, Italy
e-mail: giulia.caraceni90@gmail.com

M. Montorsi
Department of Biomedical Sciences, Humanitas University, Pieve Emanuele, Milan, Italy
Department of General Surgery, Humanitas Clinical and Research Center IRCCS, Rozzano, Milan, Italy
e-mail: marco.montorsi@hunimed.eu

A. Zerbi (✉)
Pancreatic Surgery Unit, Humanitas Clinical and Research Center IRCCS, Rozzano, Milan, Italy
Department of Biomedical Sciences, Humanitas University, Pieve Emanuele, Milan, Italy
e-mail: alessandro.zerbi@hunimed.eu

© Springer Nature Switzerland AG 2021
M. Montorsi (ed.), *Volume-Outcome Relationship in Oncological Surgery*,
Updates in Surgery, https://doi.org/10.1007/978-3-030-51806-6_6

hospitals are able to provide the highest standards of care for pancreatic surgery, and to develop specific surgical training programs for pancreatic surgeons.

The correlation between hospital volume and postoperative outcomes in pancreatic surgery has been widely demonstrated. This finding has led to the development of centralization policies to favor complex surgical procedures in high-volume hospitals. High-volume surgery and favorable outcomes have a two-way relationship. High-volume hospitals have likely implemented processes and systems of care that mediate observed volume-outcomes benefits, so that more patients are generally referred to these hospitals [3]. A study by El Amrani et al. [4] has recently shown that only a slight difference exists among high- and low-volume hospitals in terms of major postoperative complications. Conversely, the mortality is significantly higher in low-volume centers due to a failure to rescue patients with major complications. The concept of "failure to rescue" is related to ineffective management of postoperative complications, which may be considered an indicator for quality of care improvements following a high-risk surgical procedure. In addition, outcomes are generally dependent on both hospital factors (e.g., anesthesia support and intensive care) and surgeon factors (e.g., operative technique). The surgeon's expertise and case volume have been demonstrated to have a significant impact on outcomes following pancreatic surgery. An Italian study by Pecorelli et al. [5] has found the optimal cut-off of 10 pancreatectomies/year to minimize the pancreatic fistula risk. Procedures performed by surgeons with lower expertise have a greater rate of postoperative pancreatic fistula compared to more expert surgeons. Interestingly, no differences have been found in terms of postoperative mortality and morbidity, suggesting that lower technical experience can be overcome by a wiser and more experienced multidisciplinary management of complications. Also, the direct supervision of an expert surgeon in the operating room is believed to improve surgical outcomes of less expert pancreatic surgeons. At least 90 procedures are needed to complete the learning curve and to perform pancreatic surgery independently with good outcomes [6].

To guarantee appropriate surgery with low postoperative morbidity and mortality rates, different centralization policies have been established in Europe and the United States, but the optimal surgical volume cut-offs for high-volume centers remains under debate. The minimum numbers of procedures per year might widely range from 10 to >100 resections in different countries [7]. In the United States, the minimal annual hospital and surgeon volume for pancreatic surgery are 20 and 10 pancreatic resections, respectively [8–10]. In Italy, an expert consensus paper has set the minimal requirement for high-volume centers at 50 procedures every 3 years with a mortality rate less than 5% [11]. Finally, the centralization of pancreatic patients in high-volume hospitals is not only safe, but also cost-effective and therefore many countries are interested in pursuing this policy [12, 13]. However, compared to the United States, in Europe only a few countries have succeeded in the effective centralization of pancreatic surgery to specialized hospitals [10]. A possible explanation is that the health systems are very different among European countries. Each country has peculiar laws, limitations, and hurdles that affect health-system organization. For example, in Germany and France some structural limitations exist, such as an inappropriate distribution of high-volume centers. In Finland the low-density population forces patients to search high-level medical care far away from their homes or families. Conversely, the UK and the Netherlands were able to reach the highest level of centralization among European countries, thanks to a strict central definition of the volume thresholds for pancreatic surgery.

As an alternative to centralization policies, in Italy two different models, both based on the decentralization of expertise to a low-volume hospital, have been proposed with the aim of improving hospital surgical outcomes. This idea is based on the fact that it is possible to identify specific quality practices of high-volume centers, and that their "exportation" to other centers can improve their outcomes, independent of procedure volume.

The first model is based on the decentralization of a pancreatic surgeon trained in the high-volume center. A study by Capretti et al. [14] analyzed the surgical outcomes of seven Italian hospitals that shared the presence of at least one pancreatic surgeon trained under the same mentor (Prof. Di Carlo, San Raffaele Hospital, Milan) and each with a portfolio of at least 95 (range: 67–132) pancreatic procedures. Although these centers differed in terms of surgical volume, no differences in rates of major postoperative complications, pancreatic fistula, or postoperative mortality were observed between high- and low-volume hospitals. This result suggests that an expert pancreatic surgeon might be able to reduce the gap between low- and high-volume centers, as long as the minimal requisites to perform pancreatic surgery safely are guaranteed, such as the presence of an emergency department, interventional radiology and endoscopy services.

The second model is the "partnership model", based on the cooperation between two hospitals with different volumes. An example of this approach has been provided by the collaboration between the low-volume center Infermi Hospital (Rimini, Italy) and the high-volume center Humanitas Research Hospital (Rozzano, Milan, Italy) [15]. During a study period of 3 years, an expert surgeon from Humanitas Research Hospital was actively involved in the pre-, intra- and postoperative management of patients undergoing pancreatic surgery at the low-volume center. As result of this management, the overall postoperative outcomes improved greatly, and the mortality rate was significantly reduced. A possible explanation is that this approach favored a better patient selection and a reduction of unnecessary interventions. At the same time, the collaboration promoted the improvement of the surgical technique and of the management of postoperative complications, reducing the rate of failure to rescue.

6.2 Pancreatic Surgery in Italy: Relationship Between Volume and Outcome

Since 2008 the outcomes of pancreatic surgery in Italy has have described by some nationwide studies. These studies relied on the database of the Italian Ministry of Health, which includes every inpatient discharge from all public and private hospitals in Italy.

The first article was published in 2008 [16] and confirmed also for Italy what had been previously described in other countries: a direct relationship between the hospital's experience (the volume) and the mortality rates. Facilities performing ≤5 pancreaticoduodenectomies/year had a five-fold increased mortality risk in comparison with hospitals performing 80–100 pancreaticoduodenectomies/year (12.4% vs 2.6%) (Fig. 6.1).

A second study, focusing on the surgical treatment of pancreatic cancer in the period 2010–2012, was published in 2016 [17]. It showed that 89% of Italian hospitals providing surgery for pancreatic cancer belonged to the very low- or low-volume categories, with serious clinical consequences for patients and relevant excess cost for the National Health System (NHS). The study highlighted several aspects of the inadequacy of pancreatic cancer surgery when performed in low-volume hospitals:

1. *An overuse of palliative and exploratory operations for pancreatic cancer in low-volume hospitals.* Low-volume hospitals had a different surgical approach to pancreatic cancer patients, characterized by an overuse of non-resective surgery. The rate of non-resective surgery decreased progressively with increasing hospital volume, from 62.5% in very low-volume hospitals to 24.4% in very high-volume hospitals (Fig. 6.2). Multivariate analysis confirmed the independent effect of hospital volume on the type of surgery carried out (resective or non-resective): the probability of undergoing non-resective surgery was increased five-fold (adjusted odds ratio: 5.175) when patients were operated in very low-volume hospitals compared with very high-volume facilities.
2. *A higher mortality rate in cases of resection.* The volume-outcome relation of resective surgery was confirmed also in this study; overall mean mortality was 6.7%, ranging from 11.7 to 3.8%, according to the increasing volume category.

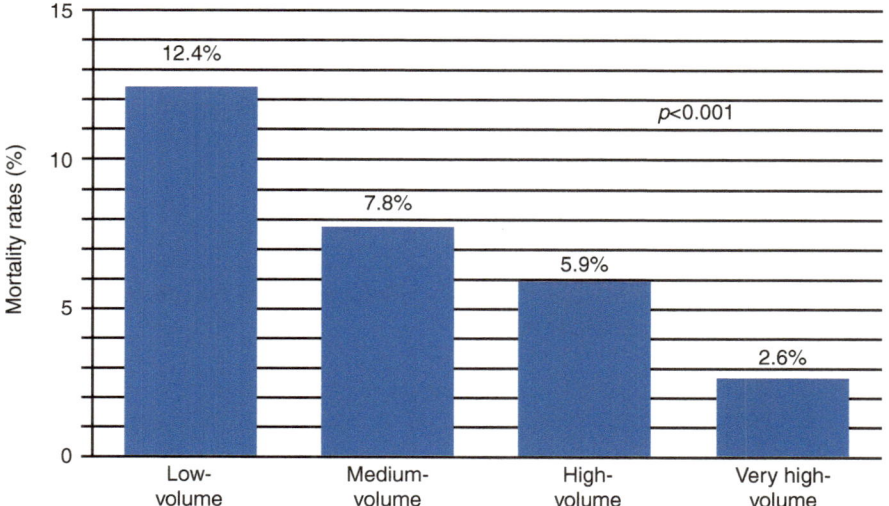

Fig. 6.1 Mortality rates after 1576 pancreaticoduodenectomies according to hospital volume

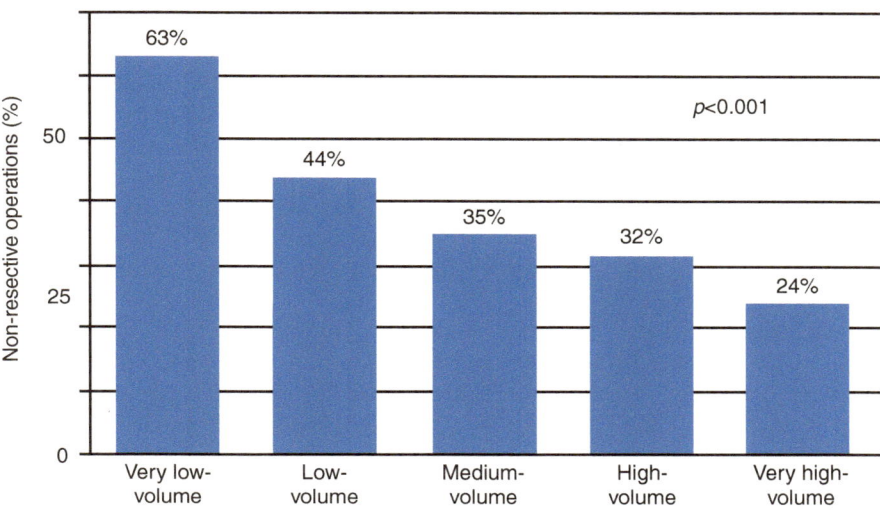

Fig. 6.2 Variability of the surgical approach to pancreatic cancer patients in different volume categories: percentage of patients undergoing non-resective operations according to hospital volume

3. *A higher mortality rate was also recorded in cases of non-resective surgery (palliative and explorative), not only for resections.* The operative mortality rate was inversely related to hospital volume even for non-resective surgery, declining from very low- to very high-volume hospitals (from 10.6 to 4.6%, $p < 0.001$). Multivariate analysis confirmed the independent effect of hospital volume on operative mortality, for both resective and non-resective surgery.
4. *An excess cost for the NHS deriving from incorrect surgery.* The estimation of avoidable costs due to the overuse of non-resective surgery in low-volume hospitals showed that more than 9.5 million euros could have been saved by the Italian NHS over a 3-year period.

A more recent study investigated resections performed between 2014 and 2016 (manuscript submitted in October 2019). The main objective of the study was the analysis of operative mortality recorded in Italian hospitals for overall pancreatic resections, evaluating both the relationship between mortality and hospital volume, and the mortality in each single hospital. Further, the outcome of operations performed in Northern, Central and Southern Italy was evaluated, and the effect of patient mobility on outcome was assessed. Of the hospitals, 305 (77%) belonged to the very low-volume category (mean 2.6 resections/year), 52 to the low-volume category (15.6 resections/year), 26 to the medium-volume category (35.9 resections/year), 8 to the high-volume category (92.7 resections/year), 4 to the very high-volume category (236.3 resections/year). In-hospital mortality for pancreatic resections was 6.1% on a national basis. A strong volume/mortality relation was confirmed: overall mortality progressively increased from 3.1% in very high-volume hospitals to 10.6% of very low-volume hospitals ($p < 0.001$). For pancreaticoduodenectomy mortality ranged from 3.4% of very high-volume hospitals to 12.3% of very low-volume hospitals ($p < 0.001$). When looking at the mortality rates of individual facilities, a great variability among hospitals belonging to the same volume group was recorded. For this analysis, centers performing less than 10 resections/year were excluded, since the number of cases would be too low to reliably reflect the actual hospital performance. This analysis included 92 hospitals with a minimal annual volume of 10 resections/year (23.3% of hospitals). The observed mortality rates of such hospitals, in relation to their annual volume of resections, are shown in Fig. 6.3.

Operative mortality was higher than 5% in 48/92 centers (52.2%), 17 of which had >10% mortality (in four centers mortality was $\geq 20\%$). Increased death rates were recorded even in some of the 38 hospitals performing ≥ 25 resections per year: mortality was >5% in 17 facilities (44.7%), five of them belonging to high- or very high-volume groups. Death rates were higher than 10% in six facilities with volume between 25 and 41 resections/year. A worrying, heterogeneous picture was derived also from the analysis of the operative mortality recorded in different geographical areas and in the individual Regions: overall mortality was higher in Southern Italy in comparison with Central and Northern Italy (10.3%, 6.6% and 5.0%, respectively ($p < 0.001$). The analysis of mortality in each single Region, showed a great variability ranging from 3.0% in Veneto to 16% in Campania (Table 6.1). Searching for high-volume hospitals, a great patient mobility was recorded: 1381 out of 3363 (41%) patients residing in Southern Italy moved to Northern (1085; 78.5%) or Central Italy (296; 21.5%) to receive pancreatic surgery. There was also a moderate mobility of patients living in Central Italy to Northern Italy (14.1%; 377 of 2663 patients). Most patients travelling for surgery (75.5%) were operated on in high- or very high-volume hospitals. Thanks to this referral, patient mobility allowed a significant reduction in mortality of Southern Italian patients: mortality was 10.4% for patients living and receiving surgery in Southern Italy and 2.7% for patients moving to Northern or Central Italy ($p < 0.001$).

6.3   Proposals for a Centralization Policy

The Italian NHS is organized on a regional basis. The central State has the task of defining the essential levels of care that must be ensured throughout the country and to monitor their actual achievement. Each Region plans and manages healthcare in full autonomy. In relation to pancreatic surgery, Italy does not provide for centralization on a national basis, and only a strict minority of Regions (Piedmont, Emilia-Romagna, Tuscany, and the Autonomous Province of Alto Adige/Südtirol), has ruled on the matter, so that virtually every hospital is authorized to perform pancreatic operations, irrespective of volume or operative mortality.

The creation of the breast units in breast cancer care should act as a model in other surgical settings, where the complexity and the need for improvement are even more relevant than in breast surgery, such as the pancreatic surgery setting. The

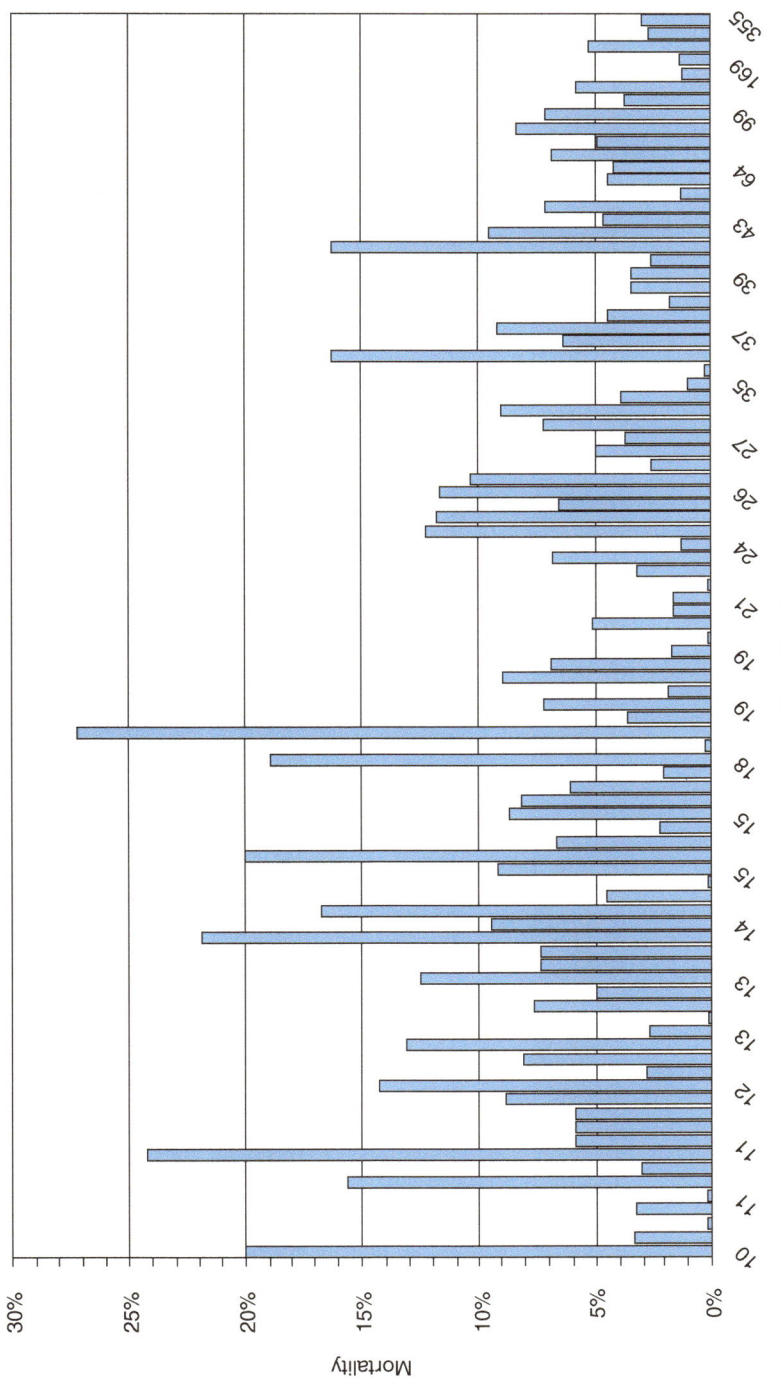

Fig. 6.3 Mortality rates after pancreatic resections in 92 Italian hospitals with a minimal volume of 10 resections/year, according to hospital volume

Table 6.1 Operative mortality after pancreatic resections in Italian Regions: period 2014–2016

Region	Mortality rate (%)	N. of resections
Piedmont	6.9	897
Lombardy	5.0	3035
Trentino-Alto Adige	3.6	165
Veneto	3.0	2275
Friuli Venezia Giulia	4.0	226
Liguria	12.6	261
Emilia-Romagna	6.5	1152
Tuscany	7.3	1096
Umbria	7.4	176
Marche	5.0	282
Lazio	6.9	1075
Abruzzo	7.7	154
Campania	16	468
Puglia	8.5	475
Basilicata	12.5	56
Calabria	9.9	71
Sicily	8.1	542
Sardinia	5.7	187

Valle d'Aosta and Molise were not included because of the low number of resections

guidelines on breast surgery, approved in 2014 by the State-Regions conference, require that each breast unit must treat at least 150 new cases per year. The data on pancreatic surgery in Italy indicate that more than 400 hospitals perform only 1–2 pancreatic cancer resections a year or even only non-resective operations [16]. When women are treated in breast units, their survival rate increases by 18%; when a patient undergoes pancreatic resection in a very-low-volume center, the risk of operative mortality increases by 300%.

In the last unpublished study, different centralization hypotheses were tested, based on the analysis of the operations performed in the period 2014–2016. As clearly described in Fig. 6.3, the outcome analysis of each hospital showed that a high surgical volume could not guarantee low mortality in all centers, although it did increase the odds of a low mortality. Therefore, without considering a mortality threshold, a hospital selection based solely on surgical volume could prove inadequate, and some centers would receive accreditation, despite having >10%, or even >20% mortality.

In our centralization simulations, a minimal volume requirement was applied either as the sole criterion, or in combination with a mortality threshold. In case of applying a mortality threshold, facilities with death rates above a determined limit would be excluded, despite meeting the volume requirement. Two minimal volume thresholds were considered: ≥10 resections/year and ≥25 resections/year. The lower cutoff was chosen since it was the lowest among the various minimal volume requirements indicated by centralization policies in North America and Europe [8]. The higher was suggested by a French national study as one of the ideal thresholds to select facilities with low mortality [18]. Two maximal mortality thresholds were then combined with the volume requirements: ≤5% and ≤10%. The results of the

Table 6.2 Comparison of the present Italian situation (no centralization policy on a national basis), with different hypotheses of centralization, based on different minimal volume requirement and different mortality thresholds

Minimal volume (resections per year)	Mortality threshold	N. of hospitals	Operative mortality in hospital selection		Patients operated in hospital selection		p-value*
			%	N. of deaths	%	N. of patients	
None	None	395	6.1	789	100.0	12,844	–
≥10	None	92	5.3	544	80.6	10,349	0.004
	≤5%	44	2.6	161	47.6	6116	<0.001
	≤10%	75	4.1	387	72.9	9368	<0.001
≥25	None	38	4.7	367	61.2	7859	<0.001
	≤5%	21	2.8	141	39.0	5015	<0.001
	≤10%	33	4.1	303	61.8	7396	<0.001

* p-value refers to the comparison between the present mortality rate and the mortality rate obtained in each hypothesis

simulations are shown in Table 6.2. All hypotheses would provide a significant improvement of mortality rates with respect to 6.1% of the present situation (range 2.6–5.3%). When considering the minimal volume as the sole parameter, if the requirement was set at ≥10 resections/year, operative mortality would be 5.3% in 92 selected hospital; if the requirement was set at ≥25 resections/year, mortality would be 4.7% in 38 selected hospitals. The exclusion of facilities with death rates >5% or >10% would allow a marked mortality reduction: the best performance in terms of mortality (2.6%) would be obtained by a combination of a minimal volume of ≥10 resections/year and a mortality threshold of ≤5%: this hypothesis would select 44 hospitals. If the mortality threshold was set at ≤10%, the overall mortality would be 4.1%, with 75 facilities included in the selection.

Basing a centralization policy on individual hospital outcomes, instead of applying the sole volume criterion, could make these measures acceptable by all surgeons and facilities: to be judged by its own results, rather than being excluded by an arbitrary judgement (the volume), will remove an understandable obstacle to centralization. The performance of each hospital can be easily measured by existing administrative data, and every year it can be updated. This allows a constant audit of hospital outcomes, with the possibility to make adjustments, if the outcome worsens.

In the Italian context, each Region should actually define its own centralization policy, considering the regional population and the geographical conformation. The actual needs of each Region should define the minimal volume thresholds to reach the best outcomes in only a few centers, in which pancreatic surgery should be centralized.

In our country, the process should pass through the center's accreditation, certified by the General Directorate of every Italian Region, according to some interdisciplinary facilities. This should be supported by training courses certified by national scientific societies that provide both "ad hoc" teaching (specialization courses, masters etc.) and the decentralization of experienced surgeons through the guarantee of a "hub and spoke" relationship able to plan the progressive acquisition of experience in harmony with a homogeneous distribution of the accredited reference centers on the national territory. It is certainly a long path and not a simple one, but it is the only one that, maintaining due respect for the professionalism of the general surgeon, could guarantee the safety and centrality of the patient as a person.

References

1. Greenblatt DY, Kelly KJ, Rajamanickam V, et al. Preoperative factors predict perioperative morbidity and mortality after pancreaticoduodenectomy. Ann Surg Oncol. 2011;18(8):2126–35.
2. Niedergethmann M, Farag Soliman M, Post S. Postoperative complications of pancreatic cancer surgery. Minerva Chir. 2004;59(2):175–83.
3. Birkmeyer JD, Finlayson SR, Tosteson AN, et al. Effect of hospital volume on in-hospital mortality with pancreaticoduodenectomy. Surgery. 1999;125(3):250–6.
4. El Amrani M, Clement G, Lenne X, et al. Failure to rescue in patients undergoing pancreatectomy: is hospital volume a standard of quality improvement programs? Nationwide analysis of 12,333 patients. Ann Surg. 2018;268(5):799–807.
5. Pecorelli N, Balzano G, Capretti G, et al. Effect of surgeon volume on outcome following pancreaticoduodenectomy in a high-volume hospital. J Gastrointest Surg. 2012;16(3):518–23.
6. Krautz C, Haase E, Elshafei M, et al. The impact of surgical experience and frequency of practice on perioperative outcomes in pancreatic surgery. BMC Surg. 2019;19(1):108. https://doi.org/10.1186/s12893-019-0577-6.
7. Vonlanthen R, Lodge P, Barkun JS, et al. Toward a consensus on centralization in surgery. Ann Surg. 2018;268(5):712–24.
8. Milstein A, Galvin RS, Delbanco SF, et al. Improving the safety of health care: the leapfrog initiative. Eff Clin Pract. 2000;3(6):313–6.
9. Finks JF, Osborne NH, Birkmeyer JD. Trends in hospital volume and operative mortality for high-risk surgery. N Engl J Med. 2011;364(22):2128–37.
10. Polonski A, Izbicki JR, Uzunoglu FG. Centralization of pancreatic surgery in Europe. J Gastrointest Surg. 2019;23(10):2081–92.
11. Bassi C, Balzano G, Zerbi A, Ramera M. Pancreatic surgery in Italy. Criteria to identify the hospital units and the tertiary referral centers entitled to perform it. Updat Surg. 2016;68(2):117–22.
12. Tran TB, Dua MM, Worhunsky DJ, et al. An economic analysis of pancreaticoduodenectomy: should costs drive consumer decisions? Am J Surg. 2016;211(6):991–7.
13. Ahola R, Sand J, Laukkarinen J. Pancreatic resections are not only safest but also most cost-effective when performed in a high-volume centre: A Finnish register study. Pancreatology. 2019;19(5):769–74.
14. Capretti G, Balzano G, Gianotti L, et al. Management and outcomes of pancreatic resections performed in high-volume referral and low-volume community hospitals lead by surgeons who shared the same mentor: the importance of training. Dig Surg. 2018;35(1):42–8.
15. Ravaioli M, Pinna AD, Francioni G, et al. A partnership model between high- and low-volume hospitals to improve results in hepatobiliary pancreatic surgery. Ann Surg. 2014;260(5):871–5; discussion 875–7.
16. Balzano G, Zerbi A, Capretti G, et al. Effect of hospital volume on outcome of pancreaticoduodenectomy in Italy. Br J Surg. 2008;95(3):357–62.
17. Balzano G, Capretti G, Callea G, et al. Overuse of surgery in patients with pancreatic cancer. A nationwide analysis in Italy. HPB (Oxford). 2016;18(5):470–8.
18. Farges O, Bendersky N, Truant S, et al. The theory and practice of pancreatic surgery in France. Ann Surg. 2017;266(5):797–804.

Volume-Outcome Relationship in Colorectal Surgery

7

Mario Morino, Antonino Spinelli, and Marco E. Allaix

7.1 Introduction

There is increasing evidence suggesting that hospital volume has a major impact on both perioperative and long-term outcomes after complex surgery for cancer [1–7]. The well-established relationship between hospital volume and outcomes in patients undergoing pancreatectomy, esophagectomy, gastrectomy and hepatectomy has led to the centralization of these complex procedures in high-volume hospitals in several countries.

The effect of volume on the outcomes of patients undergoing colorectal resection for cancer is much more debated. Even though rectal resection with total mesorectal excision (TME) for cancer is a challenging surgical procedure that is associated with significant postoperative morbidity and mortality and the treatment is frequently multimodal, the current evidence about the benefits of centralizing rectal cancer patients remains controversial. The evidence supporting the centralization of colon cancer patients is even weaker [8].

There are several factors that may be responsible for the lack of consensus on centralization policies for colon cancer surgery.

- *First*, colorectal cancer is currently the third most common cancer in men and the second in women, with an overall estimated 1,360,000 new cases in 2012. The incidence of colorectal cancer is significantly higher than that of gastric cancer,

M. Morino (✉) · M. E. Allaix
Department of Surgical Sciences, University of Turin, Turin, Italy
e-mail: mario.morino@unito.it; marcoettore.allaix@unito.it

A. Spinelli
Department of Biomedical Sciences, Humanitas University, Pieve Emanuele, Milan, Italy

Colon and Rectal Surgery Division, Humanitas Clinical and Research Center IRCCS, Rozzano, Milan, Italy
e-mail: antoninospinelli@gmail.com

© Springer Nature Switzerland AG 2021
M. Montorsi (ed.), *Volume-Outcome Relationship in Oncological Surgery*,
Updates in Surgery, https://doi.org/10.1007/978-3-030-51806-6_7

pancreatic cancer or esophageal cancer, thus making the process of centralization very challenging worldwide.

- *Second*, colon cancer has several clinical presentations, which still in 2019 require emergent surgery in local community hospitals in up to 15% of cases [9], mainly due to bowel obstruction and perforation.
- *Third*, while pancreatic or esophageal cancer surgeries are burdened by high rates of challenging complications that need a multidisciplinary treatment, involving amongst others intensivists, endoscopists, and radiologists, this is rarely the case after colectomy, with most complications being treated surgically.
- *Fourth*, patients suffering from colon cancer are infrequently discussed at multidisciplinary team meetings in referral centers. In addition, a colon resection is usually less technically demanding than rectal resection with TME or other abdominal cancer operations.

As a consequence, most colon cancer patients receive surgical treatment at the hospital where the diagnosis has been made, regardless of the caseload. However, some recent data have shown that the subgroup of patients with locally advanced colon cancer might benefit from centralization of care in referral centers [10].

The aim of this chapter is to critically revise the current evidence about the impact of volumes on the outcomes of patients with locally advanced colon cancer and rectal cancer.

7.2   Volumes and Colorectal Cancer: Current Practice and Outcome Evaluation

During the last 40 years, major efforts have been made to improve outcomes in patients undergoing colorectal surgery for cancer. For instance, the adoption of new techniques, such as laparoscopy and TME, has led to significant improvement in both short-term and long-term oncologic outcomes [11].

Along with these technical advances, the centralization of surgical care has gained increasing attention. The first article that described a relationship between surgical volume and postoperative mortality was published by Luft et al. [12] over 40 years ago. They analyzed the possible relationship between mortality and hospital's surgical volume for several surgical operations of different complexity. Mortality was 25–40% lower after complex surgery, including open-heart surgery, vascular surgery, and coronary bypass in those hospitals where 200 or more of those surgical procedures were performed each year. Other procedures, such as cholecystectomy, did not show significant relationships between volume and postoperative mortality. Similar results were obtained by Birkmeyer et al. [1] in 2002 in the United States. They evaluated the mortality rates after six different cardiovascular procedures and eight major cancer resections between 1994 and 1999, including a total of 2.5 million procedures. Mortality rates decreased by increasing the hospital volume for all 14 types of surgical operations. However, the clinical impact of the volume varied markedly according to the type of procedure. While the difference in mortality between very low-volume hospitals and very high-volume hospitals was higher than 12% for pancreatic surgery, and 5% for esophagectomy, it was less than 2% for colectomy. Similar results were observed by Hannan et al. [13]. They investigated the relationship between volume and postoperative in-hospital mortality. More than 32,000 patients undergoing colectomy, lung lobectomy, or gastrectomy for cancer between January 1, 1994 and December 31, 1997 were analyzed. Even though most benefits were obtained in gastric cancer patients, a 1.9% decrease in mortality was detected in colon cancer patients treated by high-volume surgeons. Interestingly, the relationship between volume and outcomes did not change over time, even though significant improvements occurred in surgical techniques, intensive care and patient safety. The analysis of 3,282,127 Medicare patients undergoing surgery between 2000 and 2009 confirmed that higher volume hospitals have significantly lower mortality rates than lower volume hospitals [14].

During the last 20 years, many studies have been focused on the impact of the centralization of surgery in colorectal surgery in and outside the United States, reporting controversial results (Table 7.1) [15–21]. A Cochrane review [16] was conducted in 2012 to evaluate the presence and impact of the volume-outcomes relationship and the role of specialization on both short-term and oncologic outcomes in colorectal surgery starting in 1990.

For colon cancer patients, both 5-year survival and operative mortality were not associated with hospital volume. The effect of surgeon volume was significant in terms of operative mortality, while no relevant differences were observed in long-term survival. At that time, there was very limited evidence about the incidence of postoperative anastomotic leaks based on surgeon and hospital volumes. Lastly, no conclusions on the effect of surgeon specialization were drawn due the paucity of studies focused on this topic.

For rectal cancer patients, hospital high volume was associated with better 5-year survival, while no association was observed for operative mortality. Regarding surgeon volume, significantly better results were observed only in studies with unadjusted data, while the analysis of studies using case-mix adjustment did not reveal any significant relationship. As was the case with colon cancer, the interpretation of the impact of surgeon specialization on outcomes was strongly limited by the poor quality of the available evidence. The anastomotic leak rate was significantly associated with hospital volume, but not with surgeon volume or specialization. Lastly, the rates of permanent stoma and abdominoperineal resections were significantly lower in higher volume hospitals and in patients treated by specialists and high-volume surgeons.

Very recently, an updated systematic review and meta-analysis of the literature [17] analyzed the association between hospital/surgeon volumes and outcomes. A total of 47 papers published between 1997 and 2015 were pooled together, including 1,122,303 patients, 9877 hospitals and 9649 surgeons. Thirty-day mortality was significantly lower in high-volume hospitals, while the effect of surgeon caseload was limited to colon cancer patients. Hospital and surgeon caseload did not significantly influence overall postoperative morbidity. Overall anastomotic leak rate after rectal surgery was the only complication influenced by surgeon volume and hospital

Table 7.1 Influence of hospital and surgeon volume on the outcomes of patients following colorectal cancer surgery (data from the literature)

Authors	Colon/rectum	Number of patients	30-day mortality		Overall morbidity		Anastomotic leak		Long-term survival		Local recurrence	
			HV	SV	HV	SV	HV	SV	HV	SV	HV	SV
Karanicolas et al. [15]	Colon + rectum	21,074	=	+	NE	NE	NE	NE	NE	NE	NE	NE
Huo et al. [17]	Colon	331,952	+	+	=	=	=	=	=	+	=	=
	Rectum	58,568	+	+	=	=	+	+	=	+	+	+
Buurma et al. [18]	Colon + rectum	774	NE		NE	=	NE	=	NE	+	NE	NE
Baek et al. [21]	Rectum	7187	+	NE	NE	NE	NE	NE	NE	NE	NE	NE
Burns et al. [19]	Colon + rectum	109,261	=	=	=	=	=	=	NE	NE	NE	NE
Aquina et al. [20]	Rectum	7798	+	+	NE	NE	NE	NE	NE	NE	NE	NE
Sheetz et al. [31]	Colon	4390	=	NE	=	NE	NE	NE	NE	NE	NE	NE
El Amrani et al. [28]	Rectum	45,569	+	NE	+	NE	=	NE	NE	NE	NE	NE

+ volume influence, = no volume influence, *HV* hospital volume, *SV* surgeon volume, *NE* not evaluated volume. No differences were detected in terms of anastomotic leak after colon resection. Overall, surgeon volume was associated with significantly shorter operative time and hospital stay, lower costs, greater number of lymph nodes harvested in the specimen, lower relapse rates and better 5-year survival.

The results of these reviews seem to suggest that high volumes and specializations play a key role in determining outcomes in colon and rectal cancer patients. However, the interpretation of these conclusions is challenged and biased by several factors. First, there was no agreed definition of high volume (for either hospitals or surgeons), which was very heterogeneous, with wide ranges of volume thresholds. Second, there was no consensus on the definition of a colorectal specialist. Third, emergency and elective cases were combined in the Cochrane analysis. Emergent cases were more likely performed in hospitals with low caseload, without the facilities employed for elective surgical care, and by non-specialist surgeons. Fourth, the studies considered were conducted in countries with healthcare systems that differ largely in care delivery. Lastly, the presence of other facilities, such as multidisciplinary teams and intensive care units, was not taken into consideration. It might be that the outcomes obtained in high-volume surgical institutions more closely reflect the presence of high-standard oncological care than the volume and surgical quality *per se*. As a consequence, the critical analysis of the evidence available raised the doubt about the potential risk of moving patients from low-volume providers performing high-quality surgery to high-volume providers doing low-quality surgery.

To better define if there is any significant impact of volumes *per se* on colorectal cancer patient outcomes and if the better results are related to surgical volume or to other factors, Burns et al. [19] published in 2013 the results of an observational study including 109,262 elective colorectal resections for cancer performed in England between 2000 and 2008. Consultant surgeons and hospitals were divided into three groups (low, medium and high volume) based on their mean annual volume. Provider volume was also considered a continuous variable in a second statistical model. An increase in the median volume of consultant surgeons and hospital was observed during the study period, mainly due to the trend towards surgeon specialization and patient referral to specialized centers. High-volume surgeons more likely treated rectal cancer patients and used more frequently the laparoscopic approach. However, when volume was considered a categorical variable, the high caseload of surgeons and hospitals was associated only with shorter length of hospital stay, while no differences were observed in postoperative 30-day in-hospital mortality, readmission rates or 28-day reoperation. When volume was considered a continuous variable, no association with the study outcomes was observed. It was speculated that this lack of effects of volume on patient outcomes might depend on the tendency of operating surgeons to specialize. Interestingly, significant variations in outcomes were reported even among very high-volume consultant surgeons, with mortality rates ranging between 0 and 7.7%, reoperation rates between 0.6 and 14.2%, and readmission rates between 3.6 and 16%; mean length of operative stay ranged from 6.3 to 17.8 days. These data suggest that the increase in volumes *per se* may not be sufficient to improve the postoperative outcomes of colorectal cancer patients.

To date, it is unclear if hospital volumes are more important than surgeon volumes or vice versa. Aquina et al. [20] retrospectively reviewed 7798 patients, observing a 57% decrease in 30-day mortality among patients operated on by high-volume surgeons at high-volume hospitals compared with patients treated by low-volume surgeons in low-volume hospitals. However, no significant differences were reported for high-volume surgeons operating in low-volume hospitals or for low-volume surgeons working at high-volume hospitals. Baek et al. [21] showed lower mortality and increased sphincter-preserving procedures among patients undergoing rectal resection in high-volume facilities. Evaluation of the interaction between surgeon and hospital volume revealed that the best mortality rates and oncologic outcomes were observed in high-volume hospitals with high-volume surgeons, followed by low-volume hospitals with high-volume surgeons.

Some studies have reported that low-volume hospitals with high-volume surgeons achieved better results than high-volume hospitals with low-volume surgeons, suggesting that surgeon volume is more important than hospital volumes. However, a clear threshold of effect of volumes on outcomes, and a linear relation between volume and outcomes has not been demonstrated. In addition, other factors that influence surgical outcomes are patient characteristics, including comorbidities, cancer characteristics, and surgeon characteristics, such as experience and learning curve. Regarding this latter variable, it is interesting to note that the annual volumes reported in many studies are lower than those reported in studies addressing the learning curve in colorectal surgery [22].

As also demonstrated by Kurlansky et al. [23] even low-volume hospitals with low-volume surgeons can achieve good clinical results, if the standard of evidence-based quality are followed, through multifactorial interventions, including education and periodic audit. Another possible variable that might improve outcomes after colorectal surgery is the subspecialty of surgeons in colorectal surgery. For instance, Saraidaridis et al. [24] analyzed outcomes according to colorectal training after adjusting for hospital and surgeon volume. A total of 270,684 patients undergoing surgery performed by 8217 general surgeons and 196 colorectal surgeons between 2000 and 2014 in the state of New York. Colorectal surgeons performed 26.7% of all procedures and had annual higher volumes for colectomies and proctectomies than general surgeons. Also hospital volumes were higher for the patients treated by colorectal surgeons. In-hospital mortality was significantly lower, hospital stay was significantly shorter, and a colostomy was less frequently performed in patients treated by colorectal than general surgeons. This reflects the attitude towards a more selective use of stoma and a trend towards a higher number of colorectal anastomoses. These findings support the concept that specific colorectal training provides several advantages in terms of postoperative outcomes. In the United States, colorectal subspecialty training has led to increased experience in the preoperative, intraoperative, and early postoperative management of both colon and rectal cancer patients, with particular focus on proficiency in minimally invasive laparoscopic approach. Several factors might be associated with the better outcomes observed in these patients, including the volume exposure during the training period, the specialized working setting and academic attention to this aspect. Surgeon volume goes hand in hand with the learning curve. Unfortunately, the learning curve is variable in the absence of a univocal threshold, since it depends on the outcome chosen to measure the surgeon proficiency: conversion to open surgery in the case of laparoscopic surgery, intraoperative blood loss, operative time or hospital length of stay. Several studies conducted in the United States clearly demonstrated that the mean number of laparoscopic colon resection performed over the colorectal fellowship training period was significantly higher than that performed by residents in general surgery. As a consequence, the comfort in performing laparoscopic right or left colectomy was significantly higher among specialized colorectal surgeons [25, 26].

Patient comorbidities determine the risk of postoperative mortality, regardless of hospital volume [27, 28]. In order to identify the role of hospital volume on postoperative mortality after resection according to the Charlson Comorbidity Index (CCI), El Amrani et al. [28] reviewed 45,569 rectal resections in a French nationwide study. Ninety-day postoperative mortality was 3.5% and strictly correlated to the CCI score and age. Among low-risk patients, mortality was significantly lower in high-volume hospitals (≥41 surgeries per year) than in intermediate- (10–40) or low-volume hospitals (<10) for all categories of CCI score and age. In the multivariate analysis, proctectomy in low- and intermediate-volume centers were independently associated with higher rates of postoperative mortality, along with comorbidities, open approach, anastomotic leak. Lower rates of mortality were also observed in high-volume centers among patients who experienced postoperative complications, suggesting that the ability to manage the complications in a multidisciplinary setting allows outcomes to be improved. The presence of expert interventional radiologists, endoscopists, intensive care units may be responsible for the lower rates of adverse outcomes in high-volume hospitals.

7.3 This Is the Evidence: How About Clinical Practice?

Although weak and debated, some evidence seems to suggest that the centralization of colorectal surgery might improve outcomes (Table 7.1). Nevertheless, concerns about the centralization of colorectal cancer surgery to high-volume hospitals have been raised, since it might increase disparities in the management of patients, mostly those living in rural areas and the elderly, increase the need to travel for patients and families and lead to fragmentation of postoperative care. It is important to consider that colorectal surgery includes a variety of benign, highly prevalent diseases, including diverticulitis, inflammatory bowel disease and endometriosis. The surgical skills and techniques required to treat such conditions are similar to those required to treat colorectal cancers. Therefore, centralizing oncologic colorectal surgery leads to the risk of worsening surgical results in the management of benign colorectal conditions. It has been reported that perioperative mortality significantly increases when patients are followed up at centers where the index operation was not performed and/or performed by different providers [29]. Interestingly, the implementation of rectal surgery centralization has been lower than expected even in the United States, where several studies suggesting a critical role of volume have been conducted. The "Take the Volume Pledge" (TVP) campaign was conceived in 2015 to centralize complex surgery, including esophagectomy, proctectomy and pancreatectomy [30]. Hospitals were divided in four categories, based on whether or not they met the TVP annual mean volume threshold for each surgical procedure ($\geq$15 rectal resections per year) and the total number of years each facility was considered high-volume during the study period: low-volume, intermittent low-volume, intermittent high-volume, high-volume. A retrospective cohort study of patients included in the National Cancer Data Base with a diagnosis of esophageal, pancreatic or rectal cancer was conducted. Only few US hospitals met the annual TVP threshold (high or intermittent high volume): in particular, 19.7% for proctectomy. Multimodality treatment was more likely used in high-volume than in lower volume hospitals. Similarly, the rates of positive resection margins, 30-day and 90-day mortality were all lower in the high-volume centers than in the other categories of hospitals with lower volumes. However, 48% of proctectomies were performed in low- or intermittent low-volume hospitals. Similar results were obtained by Sheetz et al. [31] who analyzed in 2019 the association between hospitals' adherence to the minimum volume standards and short-term outcomes.

The better outcomes related to the multidisciplinary approach have witnessed clinically relevant improvements during the last 10 years, mainly due to the use of MRI-based staging, use of total neoadjuvant therapy and adoption of minimally invasive approaches, including laparoscopic and robot-assisted surgery. All these developments have resulted in a significant decrease in hospital stay, severe postoperative complications rates, surgical site infections, and anastomotic leaks. Preliminary evidence seems to suggest that total neoadjuvant therapy might be associated with decreased positive circumferential margin rates and increased rates of tumor downstaging [32].

Even though population-based screening programs have been widely adopted in many countries worldwide, 10–15% of patients present with locally advanced colon or rectal cancer, with subsequent impact on management and prognosis. To date, the role of centralization of this subgroup of patients is still unclear. Indeed, very few studies have focused on the impact of volumes on the outcomes in these patients. For instance, the Dutch Surgical Colorectal Audit conducted between 2009 and 2014 and including 4980 patients with a clinical T4 colon cancer revealed that there is a very small difference in terms of number of colon resections between so-called low- and high-volume centers (2.3 vs. 6.9), suggesting that centralization has not already occurred [10]. The currently available data regarding perioperative mortality (about 6%) and recurrence rates (up to 56%), with subsequent poor survival suggest that there is room for improving outcomes in patients with locally advanced colon cancer. It has been speculated that centralization of this surgery might be associated with better results, mainly due to increased rates of multivisceral resections, minimally invasive approach and bridging strategies including decompressive stomas in cases of bowel obstruction, and implementation of neoadjuvant treatments after multidisciplinary team discussion. Recent studies [33] have shown that neoadjuvant chemo(radiation) therapy may increase the rate of R0 resections, without adding significant toxicity. However, the absence of studies with long follow-up periods does not allow any conclusion to be drawn about the oncologic impact of this strategy in locally advanced colon cancer.

Finally, volumes are interestingly not considered as a parameter in a sophisticated program like the American National Accreditation Program for Rectal Cancer (NAPRC), developed through a collaboration between the OSTRiCh (Optimizing the Surgical Treatment of Rectal Cancer) Consortium and the Commission on Cancer (CoC), a quality program of the American College of Surgeons. Indeed, the requirements for a division to qualify for such a program imply the volumes, since it is implicit that no low-volume hospital would sustain such an implementation and the related periodic auditing.

7.4 Conclusions

Even though both surgeon and hospital volume are recognized factors having a significant impact on short-term and oncologic long-term outcomes in colorectal cancer patients, surgeon expertise and caseload seem to be more crucial than hospital volumes. Indeed, hospital volume thresholds are discretionary and differences between hospitals considered low- or high-volume are diminishing over time. To date, public health policies have limited the centralization of colon and rectal cancer surgery in many countries. Furthermore, it is important not to forget the role of complex benign colorectal surgery: expertise in managing inflammatory bowel disease or diverticulitis is synergistic to oncologic colorectal surgery. As a consequence, it may be more appropriate to differentiate hospitals in high-quality and low-quality rather than in high-volume and low-volume.

References

1. Birkmeyer JD, Siewers AE, Finlayson EV, et al. Hospital volume and surgical mortality in the United States. N Engl J Med. 2002;346(15):1128–37.
2. Fong Y, Gonen M, Rubin D, Radzyner M, Brennan MF. Long-term survival is superior after resection for cancer in high-volume centers. Ann Surg. 2005;242(4):540–4; discussion 544–7.
3. Gooiker GA, van Gijn W, Wouters MW, et al. Systematic review and meta-analysis of the volume-outcome relationship in pancreatic surgery. Br J Surg. 2011;98(4):485–94.
4. Tol JA, van Gulik TM, Busch OR, Gouma DJ. Centralization of highly complex low-volume procedures in upper gastrointestinal surgery. A summary of systematic reviews and meta-analyses. Dig Surg. 2012;29(5):374–83.
5. Pasquer A, Renaud F, Hec F, et al. Is centralization needed for esophageal and gastric cancer patients with low operative risk? A nationwide study. Ann Surg. 2016;264(5):823–30.
6. Farges O, Bendersky N, Truant S, et al. The theory and practice of pancreatic surgery in France. Ann Surg. 2017;266(5):797–804.
7. Mark-Christensen A, Erichsen R, Brandsborg S, et al. Pouch failures following ileal pouch–anal anastomosis for ulcerative colitis. Color Dis. 2018;20(1):44–52.
8. Vonlanthen R, Lodge P, Barkun JS, et al. Toward a consensus on centralization in surgery. Ann Surg. 2018;268(5):712–24.

9. Wanis KN, Ott M, Van Koughnett JAM, et al. Long-term oncological outcomes following emergency resection of colon cancer. Int J Color Dis. 2018;33(11):1525–32.
10. Klaver CE, Gietelink L, Bemelman WA, et al. Locally advanced colon cancer: evaluation of current clinical practice and treatment outcomes at the population level. J Natl Compr Cancer Netw. 2017;15(2):181–90.
11. Arezzo A, Passera R, Salvai A, et al. Laparoscopy for rectal cancer is oncologically adequate: a systematic review and meta-analysis of the literature. Surg Endosc. 2015;29(2):334–48.
12. Luft HS, Bunker JP, Enthoven AC. Should operations be regionalized? The empirical relation between surgical volume and mortality. N Engl J Med. 1979;301(25):1364–9.
13. Hannan EL, Radzyner M, Rubin D, et al. The influence of hospital and surgeon volume on in-hospital mortality for colectomy, gastrectomy, and lung lobectomy in patients with cancer. Surgery. 2002;131(1):6–15.
14. Reames BN, Ghaferi AA, Birkmeyer JD, Dimick JB. Hospital volume and operative mortality in the modern era. Ann Surg. 2014;260(2):244–51.
15. Karanicolas PJ, Dubois L, Colquhoun PH, et al. The more the better?: the impact of surgeon and hospital volume on in-hospital mortality following colorectal resection. Ann Surg. 2009;249(6):954–9.
16. Archampong D, Borowski D, Wille-Jørgensen P, Iversen LH. Workload and surgeon's specialty for outcome after colorectal cancer surgery. Cochrane Database Syst Rev. 2012;3:CD005391.
17. Huo YR, Phan K, Morris DL, Liauw W. Systematic review and a meta-analysis of hospital and surgeon volume/outcome relationships in colorectal cancer surgery. J Gastrointest Oncol. 2017;8(3):534–46.
18. Buurma M, Kroon HM, Reimers MS, Neijenhuis PA. Influence of individual surgeon volume on oncological outcome of colorectal cancer surgery. Int J Surg Oncol. 2015;2015:464570. https://doi.org/10.1155/2015/464570.
19. Burns EM, Bottle A, Almoudaris AM, et al. Hierarchical multilevel analysis of increased caseload volume and postoperative outcome after elective colorectal surgery. Br J Surg. 2013;100(11):1531–8.
20. Aquina CT, Probst CP, Becerra AZ, et al. High volume improves outcomes: the argument for centralization of rectal cancer surgery. Surgery. 2016;159(3):736–48.
21. Baek JH, Alrubaie A, Guzman EA, et al. The association of hospital volume with rectal cancer surgery outcomes. Int J Color Dis. 2013;28(2):191–6.
22. Mackenzie H, Markar SR, Askari A, et al. National proficiency-gain curves for minimally invasive gastrointestinal cancer surgery. Br J Surg. 2016;103(1):88–96.
23. Kurlansky PA, Argenziano M, Dunton R, et al. Quality, not volume, determines outcome of coronary artery bypass surgery in a university-based community hospital network. J Thorac Cardiovasc Surg. 2012;143(2):287–93.
24. Saraidaridis JT, Hashimoto DA, Chang DC, et al. Colorectal surgery fellowship improves in-hospital mortality after colectomy and proctectomy irrespective of hospital and surgeon volume. J Gastrointest Surg. 2018;22(3):516–22.
25. Shanker BA, Soliman M, Williamson P, Ferrara A. Laparoscopic colorectal training gap in colorectal and surgical residents. JSLS. 2016;20(3):e2016.00024. https://doi.org/10.4293/JSLS.2016.00024.
26. Stein S, Stulberg J, Champagne B. Learning laparoscopic colectomy during colorectal residency: what does it take and how are we doing? Surg Endosc. 2012;26(2):488–92.
27. LaPar DJ, Kron IL, Jones DR, et al. Hospital procedure volume should not be used as a measure of surgical quality. Ann Surg. 2012;256(4):606–15.
28. El Amrani M, Clement G, Lenne X, et al. The impact of hospital volume and Charlson score on postoperative mortality of proctectomy for rectal cancer: a nationwide study of 45,569 patients. Ann Surg. 2018;268(5):854–60.
29. Brooke BS, Goodney PP, Kraiss LW, et al. Readmission destination and risk of mortality after major surgery: an observational cohort study. Lancet. 2015;386(9996):884–95.
30. Jacobs RC, Groth S, Farjah F, et al. Potential impact of 'take the volume pledge' on access and outcomes for gastrointestinal cancer surgery. Ann Surg. 2019;270(6):1079–89.

31. Sheetz KH, Dimick JB, Nathan H. Centralization of high-risk cancer surgery within existing hospital systems. J Clin Oncol. 2019;37(34):3234–42.
32. Roxburgh CSD, Strombom P, Lynn P, et al. Changes in the multidisciplinary management of rectal cancer from 2009 to 2015 and associated improvements in short-term outcomes. Color Dis. 2019;21(10):1140–50.
33. Cukier M, Smith AJ, Milot L, et al. Neoadjuvant chemoradiotherapy and multivisceral resection for primary locally advanced adherent colon cancer: a single institution experience. Eur J Surg Oncol. 2012;38(8):677–82.

Volume-Outcome Relationship in Surgery of Soft Tissue Sarcomas

8

Gaya Spolverato, Vittorio Quagliuolo,
and Alessandro Gronchi

8.1 Introduction

Soft tissue sarcomas (STS) are rare malignancies of the connective tissue, accounting for 1% of all tumors. The incidence of STS is 6 per 100,000 inhabitants/year, with a slight male predominance. STS are more common among the childhood cancers, representing 15% of all pediatric solid malignancies, while they are very rare in adolescents. STS include over 80 different histological entities with approximately 200 molecular subtypes. STS arise from soft tissue in 75% of cases, from gastrointestinal stroma in 15% and from bone in 10%. The most common site of origin is the extremities (50%), followed by the retroperitoneum (20%), the viscera (15%), the superficial trunk (10%) and the head and neck (5%). Sarcomas are more common in the sixth decade of life, but there are age variations depending on the different histological types (i.e., embryonal/alveolar rhabdomyosarcoma and Ewing sarcoma in pediatric patients, synovial sarcoma and myxoid liposarcoma in younger adults and leiomyosarcoma and myxofibrosarcoma in older patients) [1].

Tumor-related factors, such as age, size, grade and histology have been shown to be predictors of overall survival and are included in nomograms for sarcomas of the extremities and retroperitoneum (www.sarculator.com). However, several

G. Spolverato
Department of Surgical, Oncological and Gastroenterological Sciences,
University of Padua, Padua, Italy
e-mail: gaya.spolverato@unipd.it

V. Quagliuolo
Department of Surgery, Humanitas Clinical and Research Center IRCCS,
Rozzano, Milan, Italy
e-mail: vittorio.quagliuolo@cancercenter.humanitas.it

A. Gronchi (✉)
Sarcoma Service, Department of Surgery, Fondazione IRCCS
Istituto Nazionale dei Tumori, Milan, Italy
e-mail: alessandro.gronchi@istitutotumori.mi.it

© Springer Nature Switzerland AG 2021
M. Montorsi (ed.), *Volume-Outcome Relationship in Oncological Surgery*,
Updates in Surgery, https://doi.org/10.1007/978-3-030-51806-6_8

treatment-related factors, such as quality of surgery and use of radiotherapy and/or chemotherapy are reported to have a similar impact on prognosis. In general, local recurrence is more common among some low-grade tumors, while high-grade STS tend to spread distantly. Similarly, retroperitoneal sarcomas tend to have a local pattern of recurrence, while extremity STS favor a distant spread. Among the extremity STS, myxofibrosarcomas are more likely to recur locally, while vascular sarcoma, undifferentiated pleomorphic sarcoma, leiomyosarcoma and synovial sarcoma have a much higher risk of distant metastasis. Although the lung is usually the first metastatic site of STS, some histologic subtypes may have peculiar metastatic patterns (i.e., high-grade myxoid liposarcomas have a high tropism for the abdomen, mediastinum, soft tissues and bone).

Surgery is the only potentially curative treatment for localized STS and should consist of wide en-bloc resection of the tumor with microscopic negative margins. In particular, quality of the initial surgery is reported to be the strongest predictor of recurrence-free and overall survival. However, in order to maximize the long-term oncological outcome, surgery should be tailored to the specific histologic type and be part of a multidisciplinary management of the disease.

In general, STS patients should be managed at sarcoma centers that allow for a multidisciplinary discussion of the cases between the surgical oncologist, the medical oncologist, the radiation oncologist, the radiologist and the pathologist. Moreover, given the complexity of the surgeries, support from other specialists (i.e., plastic surgeon, vascular surgeon, urologist, and thoracic surgeon) should be warranted.

In the present chapter we discuss the complexity of the approach to sarcomas and the importance of centralization of their management in delivering the best care to sarcoma patients, still afflicted by a high rate of erroneous diagnoses and unplanned surgical excisions as well as suboptimal management at non-specialized centers.

8.2   Principles of Surgery

Sarcomas usually present as solid masses. The periphery of the lesion is the most vital part of the mass. It is generally surrounded by a pseudocapsule of variable thickness consisting of compressed tumor cells embedded in a fibrovascular tissue, rarely associated with an inflammatory component, and in continuity with the surrounding normal tissues. This is the reason why a simple excision, i.e., enucleation, cannot be curative, even if most sarcomas do not seem to infiltrate surrounding structures.

Indeed, sarcomas respect anatomical borders. Thus, the local anatomy influences tumor growth by setting natural barriers to their extension. In general, sarcomas take the path allowed by least resistance anatomical planes and initially grow within the anatomical compartment in which they arose. Only at a later stage are the walls of that compartment violated (i.e., the cortex of a bone or the aponeurosis of a muscle) and the tumor breaks into another compartment. STS may arise between compartments (thus being extracompartmental) or in anatomical sites that are not walled off by anatomical barriers, such as the intermuscular or subcutaneous planes, as well as the retroperitoneum. In the latter case, they remain extracompartmental and only at a later stage break into the adjacent compartment.

There are four basic types of excisions, depending on the relationship of the dissection plane to the surface of the tumor.

- An *intralesional excision* is performed within the tumor mass and results in removal of only a portion, so that macroscopic tumor is left behind.
- In a *marginal excision*, the dissection plane crosses the pseudocapsule of the tumor. Such an excision may leave microscopic disease, and microscopic margins may be either positive or negative, depending on the type of tumor and surrounding tissues.
- A *wide excision* entails removing the tumor with a cuff of circumferential healthy tissue. However, the adequate thickness of this cuff varies broadly according to the type of tissue. It should be of some centimeters along the longitudinal plane of the muscle. It can be 1 cm along the axial plane of the muscle. It can be few millimeters, or even less, in proximity of tissues particularly resistant to tumor, such as vascular adventitia, periosteum, epineurium, peritoneum, or pleura. If not infiltrated, the underlying structures can be safely preserved. If infiltrated, their removal should always be considered.
- *Radical resection* implies removal of the tumor and the whole anatomical compartment in which it is located.

The quality of surgical margins is critical and ideally should be always evaluated by both the operating surgeon and the pathologist. The closest margin should be identified and extensively sampled. Microscopically, margins are defined as negative, when the tumor edge is covered by at least 1 mm of healthy tissue, or positive when the tumor edge is covered by <1 mm of healthy tissue or is found at the inked surface.

In principle, the aim of surgery is to resect the tumor surrounded by healthy tissue and to avoid positive surgical margins [2]. In fact, the risk of local failure doubles in case of positive margins, despite the use of postoperative RT, with a subsequent impact on distant outcome and survival. While the initial prognosis mainly depends on the biology of the tumor, once a patient has 'survived' the first period and the systemic risk dependent on tumor biology becomes weaker, the quality of surgery appears as the strongest prognosticator for outcome. Two factors can explain the impact of positive surgical margins on survival: a relatively slight increase in the risk of subsequent systemic spread in case of recurrence and a direct impact of local recurrence that may lead to death in some sites. This is typically true for tumors located to the trunk (i.e., retroperitoneum). However, a positive margin can be planned in advance in order to preserve an important structure for function-sparing (i.e., a motor nerve) or reduce morbidity (i.e., duodenum/head of the pancreas), provided adequate radiotherapy and or chemotherapy are delivered in the preoperative setting. Size, site histologic subtypes as well as anatomical constraints, function preservation, postoperative morbidities and quality of life should all be factored in making decisions about the treatment strategy. This underlines the importance of the multidisciplinary approach and specific knowledge of the natural history of the different histologic subtypes.

8.2.1   Extremity and Trunk Wall STS

Until Rosenberg et al. in the early 1980s proved that the outcome of patients with high-grade extremity STS undergoing limb-sparing surgery with adjuvant radiation therapy did not differ from those treated by primary amputation, the standard treatment for extremity STS was amputation. Now the goal in extremity STS is limb-sparing and function-sparing resections, while achieving adequate surgical margins (Fig. 8.1). The necessity to cover the soft tissue loss by a flap transposition depends on several factors, such as the site and size of the defect, exposed structures (bone, vessels, nerves), and functional restoration. Vessels, nerves, and bone are always resected when directly invaded/encased, while their resection has to be discussed on a case-by-case basis when their periosteum, adventitia or epineurium are infiltrated without invasion of the underlying structure. The rates of local recurrence in the

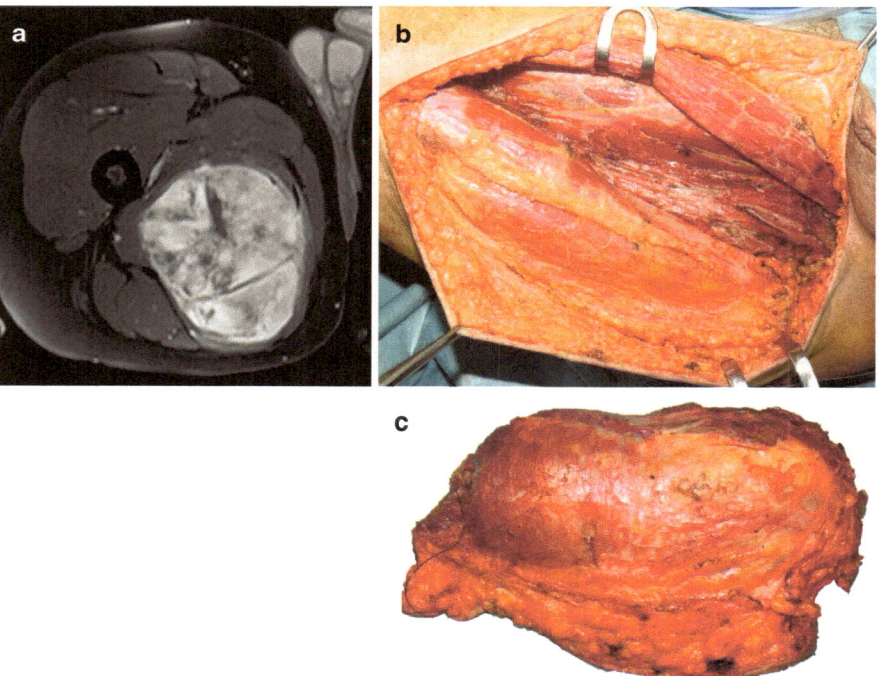

Fig. 8.1 (**a**) Axial contrast-enhanced T1-weighted magnetic resonance imaging view of a primary undifferentiated pleomorphic sarcoma of the right thigh, adductor compartment. (**b**) Surgical field after tumor removal, with evidence of a significant muscle resection. (**c**) Surgical specimen (the tumor is entirely contained in a cuff of healthy muscles)

trunk and in the extremities range between 5 and 10%, and rarely impact overall survival (OS), so that a wider resection and even amputation can be left as salvage treatment in the case of recurrent disease. Several studies evaluated the impact of margin status on the long-term outcome of patients with STS of the extremities and trunk [3]. Patients undergoing an R1 resection tend to have a higher risk of local recurrence which does not affect distant recurrence. In particular, in non-metastatic extremity and truncal STS, an R1-positive margin ≤1 mm may be adequate in the context of a multidisciplinary treatment. When close margins can be anticipated, preoperative chemotherapy/radiotherapy may be a reasonable option to maximize the chance of cure [4].

The histologic subtype should be also weighted in the decision-making process. In particular, myxofibrosarcoma has a local recurrence rate up to 30%, especially when negative margins cannot be achieved. It infiltrates through soft tissue beyond the visible or palpable mass invading into the anatomic boundaries and determining a 16% rate of distant recurrence. In addition, some histologic subtypes may be more sensitive to conventional chemotherapy (i.e., synovial sarcoma, high grade myxoid liposarcoma, undifferentiated pleomorphic sarcoma) or radiotherapy (i.e., myxoid liposarcoma) or other newer agents, such as sunitinib/pazopanib (in alveolar soft part sarcoma, extraskeletal myxoid chondrosarcoma, solitary fibrous tumor, etc.) and sirolimus/everolimus (in perivascular epithelioid cells tumors, etc.) [5].

8.2.2 Retroperitoneal STS

Retroperitoneal sarcomas (RPS) are large tumors that recur in a locoregional manner in 20–50% of patients. Local recurrence correlates with OS in the same way as distant recurrence, as patients die of inoperable locoregional disease even more frequently than of distant metastases.

Unlike primary epithelial solid tumors, which are usually confined to a single organ and can generally be removed with resection of that organ, retroperitoneal STS commonly abut multiple surrounding organs. Paralleling surgery in the extremities, tumors should be systematically resected en bloc with surrounding tissues, which at this site are mainly the adjacent viscera even when not overtly involved, to minimize the risk of microscopically positive margins (Fig. 8.2). This is particularly true for liposarcomas (well-differentiated and de-differentiated), which account for 55–60% of all RPS. Their locoregional risk is the highest among all RPS, as their well-differentiated component is virtually undistinguishable from the normal retroperitoneal fat and it is often underestimated, especially by non-specialized surgeons. Surgery often includes ipsilateral nephrectomy and colectomy; locoregional peritonectomy and myomectomy (partial/total) of the muscle of the lateral/posterior abdominal wall (usually psoas); splenectomy and left pancreatectomy for tumors located on the left upper side; occasionally pancreaticoduodenectomy or hepatectomy for tumors located on the right upper side; and vascular and bone resection only if vessels/bone are overtly infiltrated.

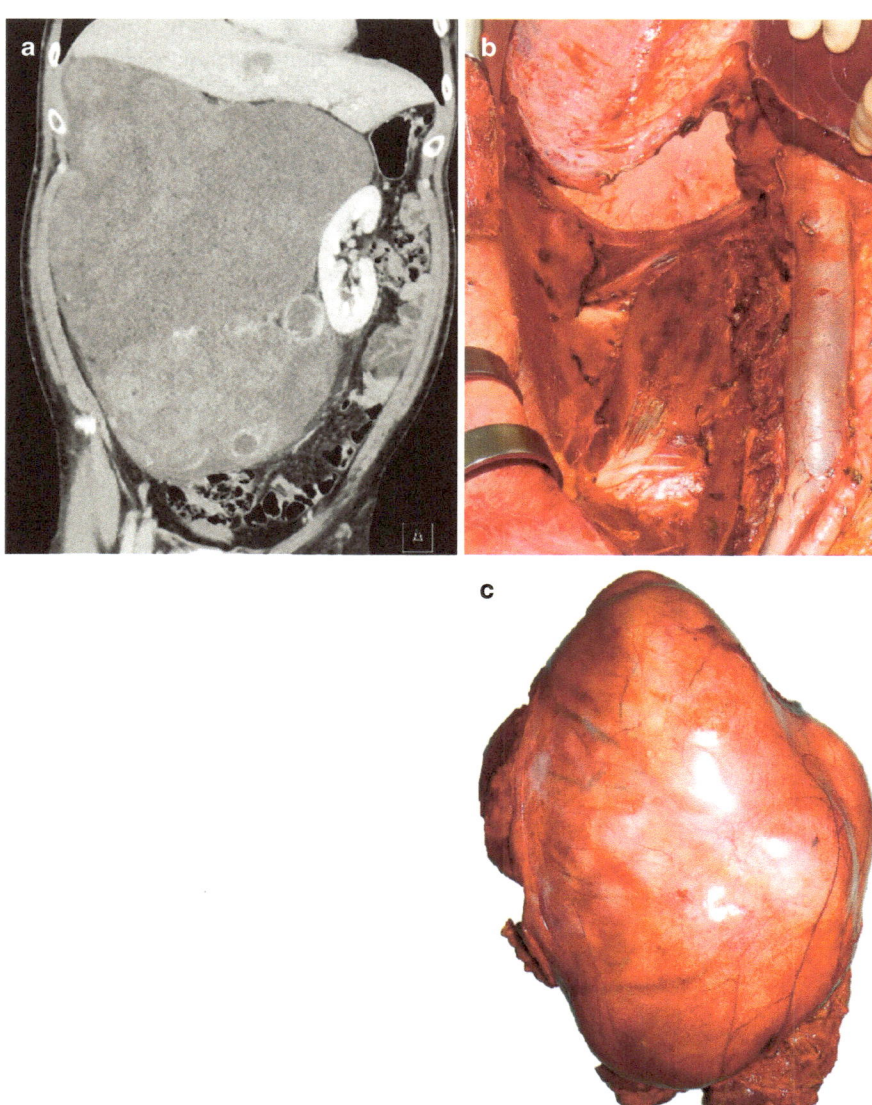

Fig. 8.2 (**a**) Coronal contrast-enhanced computed tomography portal phase scan of a primary dedifferentiated liposarcoma of the right retroperitoneum. (**b**) Surgical field after tumor removal, with evidence of removal of the tumor en-bloc with the right kidney and adrenal, right colon, right psoas muscle and a portion of the right diaphragm, while the right liver lobe is flipped contralaterally. (**c**) Surgical specimen entirely covered by the adherent viscera (right kidney and adrenal, right colon, psoas muscle, segment of diaphragm and peritoneum)

In the other retroperitoneal histologic subtypes, such as leiomyosarcoma, solitary fibrous tumor, malignant peripheral nerve sheath tumors, the approach is more variable and depends on tumor presentation and direct organ invasion. These tumors have a locoregional extension which is easier to assess. In addition, failures predominantly occur at distant sites. Surgery should still be aimed at achieving a negative margin resection. However, this can be more often achieved saving also close organs if not directly involved.

Of note, the role of surgical margins in RPS has not been established as it has been in the extremities, in part due to the challenges of pathologic assessment of the margins in large tumors and to the absence of a standardized protocol to process the specimens. While negative margin resection is the goal, pathological assessment of the status of surgical margins is usually suboptimal and not reliable in retrospective series [6].

Finally, while in extremity soft tissue sarcoma locoregional failures can always be salvaged by a surgical procedure such as an amputation, in truncal sarcoma and especially in retroperitoneal sarcoma, when locoregional failures occur, there are no salvage surgeries and the risk of death associated with an inappropriate initial resection cannot be counterbalanced by any further operation. This directly affects the chance of cure of the single patient.

8.3 Principle of Multidisciplinary Management

A multidisciplinary approach is the goal in all cases of STS. Treatment strategies for all patients must be the result of the consensus of the multidisciplinary team (MDT) including surgical oncologists, pathologists, radiologists, radiation therapists, and medical oncologists [7]. The expanded MDT includes pediatric and geriatric oncologists, nuclear medicine specialists, organ-based specialists, oncology-pharmacists, psycho-oncologists, palliative care experts, and physiotherapists. The heart of this decision-making process is a weekly MDT meeting where all patients are discussed balancing the recommendations of clinical guidelines with the complexity of the single case. In particular, the MDT meet to discuss the first diagnosis, multidisciplinary treatment, follow-up protocols, recurrent disease, deviations from clinical practice guidelines, discrepancies from histology and imaging, and options for genetic testing.

8.3.1 Diagnosis

The appropriate diagnostic assessment includes imaging, histology and molecular biology. In particular, magnetic resonance imaging (MRI) is the main imaging modality in the extremities, pelvis and trunk, while computed tomography (CT) is preferred in retroperitoneal sarcomas. In addition, staging often includes an assessment of the chest by a baseline CT scan. Multiple core needle biopsies, possibly by using 14–16 G needles, are mandatory for the diagnosis. However, an excisional biopsy may be preferred for <3 cm superficial lesions. A molecular analysis, such as fluorescence in situ hybridization for gene translocations or immunohistochemistry for aberrant protein expression, allows one to refine the diagnosis and in some instances to identify targeted agents tested in clinical trials.

8.3.2 Multidisciplinary Management of Extremity STS

Adjuvant radiation and chemotherapy both play a role in the management of extremity STS. Each STS carries its own propensity to spread locally or distantly, and nomograms predicting histology-specific rates of recurrence and survival can assist the clinician in the decision-making process. In general, tumors that tend to recur locally may benefit from radiation, whereas tumors with metastatic potential may require systemic treatment or a combination of both. Patients who benefit the most from radiation are those with large, high-grade sarcomas that carry a significant risk of local recurrence.

Identifying the ideal candidates for adjuvant or neoadjuvant chemotherapy is more difficult than those for radiation. Considering that approximately 25–50% of patients with extremity STS develop distant disease, several trials have been run in an attempt to identify the best candidates for systemic chemotherapy. In general, patients with large (>10 cm), deep, high-grade STS benefit the most from doxorubicin and ifosfamide-based chemotherapy. However, chemosensitive sarcomas, such as synovial sarcoma and high grade myxoid liposarcoma, benefit from adjuvant treatment possibly even in the context of smaller lesions. Differently, patients with chemoresistant sarcomas, such as clear cell sarcomas, alveolar soft part sarcomas and others, have classically not been prescribed conventional neoadjuvant chemotherapy. However, other agents have proven to be effective in rarer sarcomas and can be considered on an individual basis, whenever a neoadjuvant treatment is needed to maximize the chance of a complete surgical resection. Conventional chemotherapy can also be administered concurrent to radiotherapy to maximize tumor response, especially when limb/function preservation can be difficult or positive margins are expected. The same applies to trabectedin, which was recently shown to be very well tolerated in combination with radiotherapy and could become a standard approach in high-grade myxoid liposarcoma.

Hyperthermic isolated limb perfusion is an option in patients not fit for or failing other treatments, but the procedure is available at only a few specialized centers.

8.3.3 Multidisciplinary Management of Retroperitoneal Sarcomas

The role of radiation therapy in RPS is still debated. Due to the contiguity to radiosensitive organs and to the large radiation field, the use of radiotherapy for RPS is very limited. The preliminary results of STRASS-1, the first randomized, multicenter, international trial, aiming to understand the efficacy of radiotherapy combined with surgery in RPS, failed to demonstrate a benefit of preoperative radiotherapy. However, 5-year abdominal recurrence-free survival was significantly higher in well-differentiated and grade 1 or 2 dedifferentiated liposarcomas treated with preoperative radiotherapy compared to surgery alone [8].

The role of chemotherapy in RPS, mostly in high risk forms, such as G3 dedifferentiated liposarcoma and leiomyosarcoma, is debated and a new randomized trial (STRASS-2) is in preparation to analyze the role of neoadjuvant chemotherapy for high-grade liposarcoma and leiomyosarcoma of the retroperitoneum.

8.4   Centralization of Sarcoma Care

Given the complexity of the disease and the heterogeneity of the various presentations, it is intuitive that the management of sarcoma patients should be centralized to referral centers and/or within referral networks that share multidisciplinary expertise. These centers should treat a high number of patients annually and be involved in ongoing clinical trials that allow for the best tailored treatment for each specific case [9].

In general, centralization of the surgical resection of common cancers in specialized centers is advocated to minimize postoperative morbidity and mortality. However, very little is available to show an impact of centralization on the overall cure rate. In sarcomas, instead, centralization is predominantly advocated to directly impact sarcoma-specific survival. In other words, the initial multidisciplinary approach as well as the performance of the surgical resection in a specialized center have been shown to increase the cure rate. This is especially true for sarcoma of the trunk, where the cure rate increases up to 20%. Unplanned resections may indeed come at a lower postoperative morbidity risk compared to adequate wide excision. This applies at all anatomic sites, but it is even more critical in truncal sarcomas. It has also been shown that the lack of specific expertise is not compensated by compliance with guidelines.

Case volume is the inevitable first criterion to define referral centers. Different thresholds have been hypothesized. However, none of them was really supported by strong data until very recently. Most of the empirical evidence now available comes from the French National Cancer Institute clinical network for sarcoma (NETSARC) founded in 2009 and including 26 reference centers throughout the nation. In a recent study on 35,784 patients and 155 different histological subtypes of sarcoma, surgery at a NETSARC center was found to correlate with OS, local relapse-free survival, and event-free survival (Fig. 8.3) [10]. In addition, also presentation to an MDT board was associated with an improved local relapse-free survival and event-free survival, but it was an adverse prognostic factor for OS if surgery was not performed in a referral center. Taken together, these findings show how personalizing the approach to the single patient improves the cure rate [11].

Several reports have recently been published on the subgroup of retroperitoneal sarcomas, which, given the peculiarity of their presentation, cannot be salvaged by a second procedure [12–15]. One of the latest and most extensive

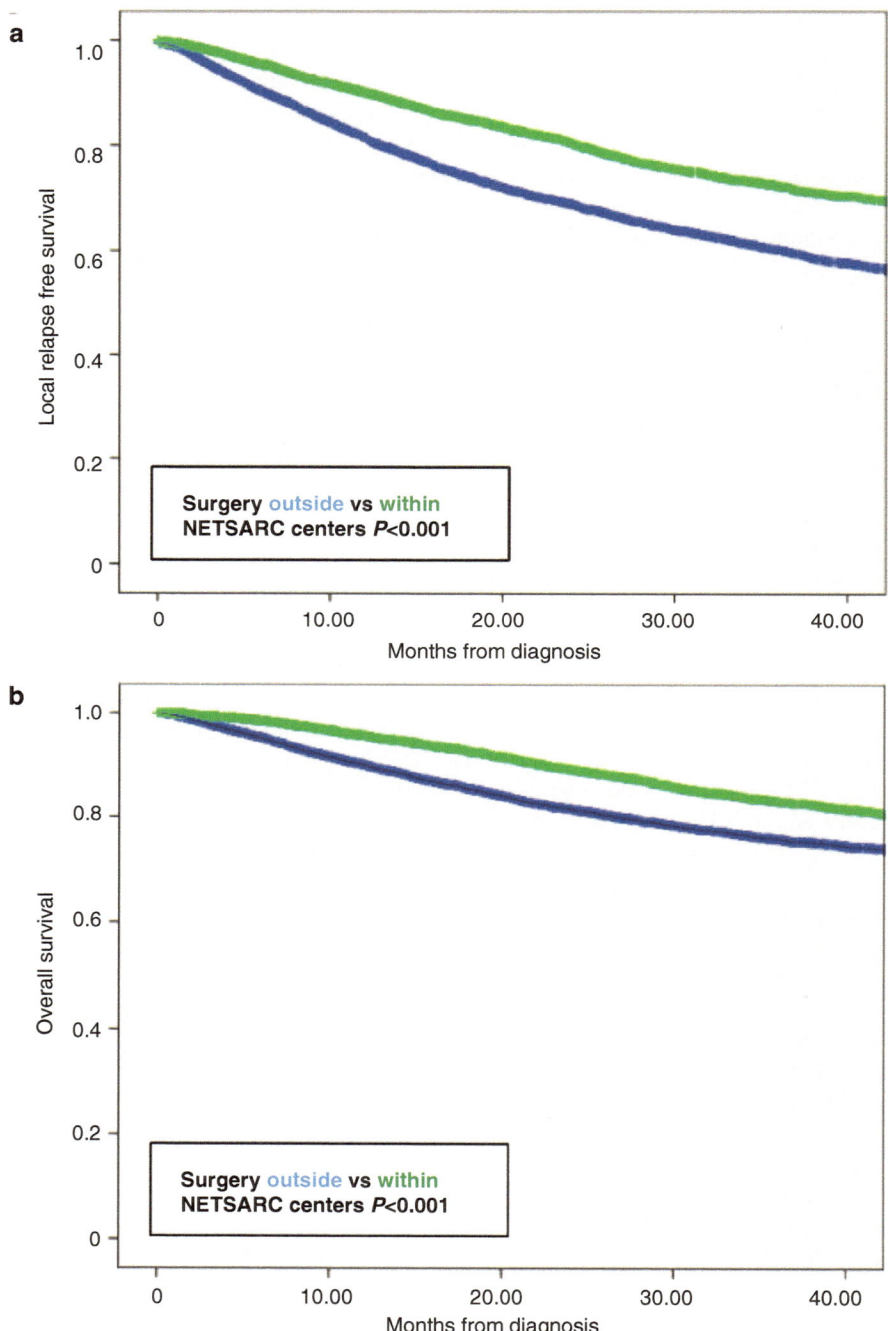

Fig. 8.3 Local relapse-free survival (**a**) and overall survival (**b**) of patients affected by soft tissue sarcoma originating at any site, surgically treated inside (*green line*) or outside (*blue line*) NETSARC centers. (Reproduced with permission from [10])

describes a cohort of 2945 patients with RPS treated in France: this report showed that two-third of surgeries were performed outside the NETSARC network (63.4% vs. 36.6%), in hospitals with a median number of surgeries of 1 (versus 23 of the NETSARC centers) [13]. The network centers showed not only higher diagnostic performance and quality of surgery, but also better long-term outcomes of patients with RPS (Fig. 8.4). In particular, the delta of 2-year

Fig. 8.4 Local relapse-free survival (**a**) and overall survival (**b**) of patients affected by soft tissue sarcoma originating from the retroperitoneum, surgically treated inside (*yellow line*) or outside (*blue line*) NETSARC centers. (Reproduced with permission from [13])

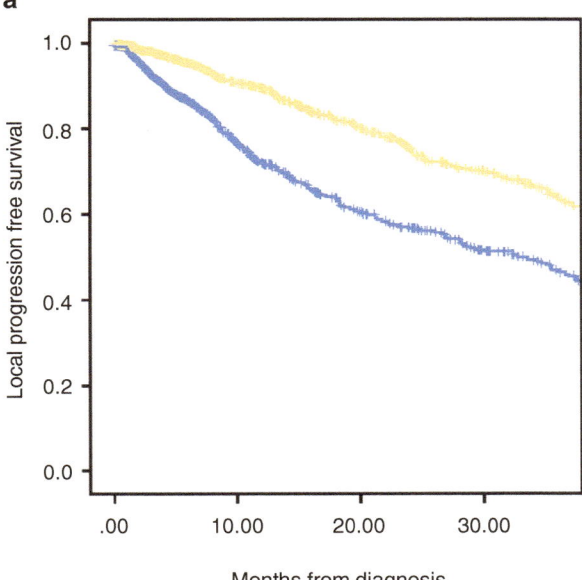

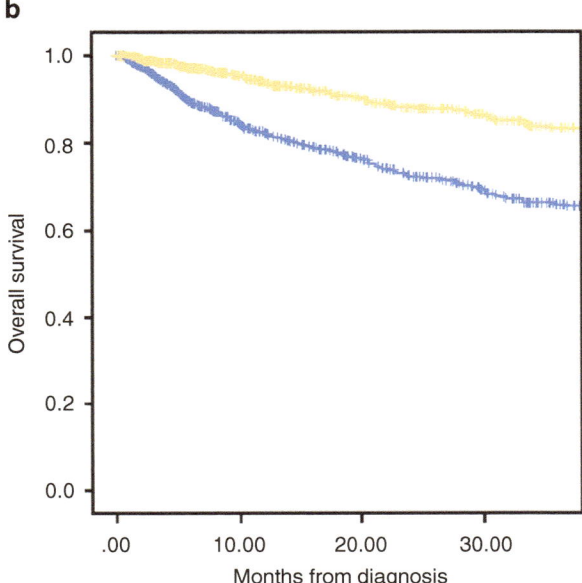

OS of patients treated inside NETSARC versus outside was 17% and the odds ratio of death was two-fold lower. The National Cancer Database, a collaborative effort of the American Cancer Society and the American College of Surgeons, was also queried in order to explore the regionalization of RPS to high-volume centers. In the United States only 9.6% of patients undergo RPS surgery at high-volume sarcoma centers. When compared to pancreatic cancer surgery, the rate of RPS regionalization grew at 30.5% of the rate of pancreatic cancer, reinforcing the call to regionalize surgery [14]. Using the same database, other authors showed that patients treated at low-volume hospitals were more likely to have lower grade and smaller tumors and undergo incomplete macroscopic resection. Differently, patients treated at high-volume centers had lower readmission rates, 30- and 90-day mortality, longer median OS and higher 5-year OS. However, the minimum procedural volume threshold is still not well defined. In detail, Keung et al. found a significant improvement in long-term OS each increment of 5 new patients per year up to >10 (Fig. 8.5) [15]. In another report based on the same data set, in a risk-adjusted survival analysis, 13 cases/year was identified as the best threshold, after which the 90-day mortality and the overall mortality did not improve further (Fig. 8.6) [16]. Of note, one of the major limitations of these two reports was that the threshold (>10 patients/year and ≥13 patients/year) was set above the 90th percentile. In other words, only 9.8% of the patients in the former and 4.4% of the patients in the latter were operated on in centers treating a number of new patients per year above the threshold. Therefore, it is not possible at this stage to define the real threshold above which there would be no further improvement in OS [17]. However, the two studies are very important because they show that patients operated on at low-volume centers are at a higher risk of death. In addition, it is also worthy of note that direct expertise can in part be substituted by working in a network. Again, the French experience with NETSARC showed how performing surgery outside the NETSARC centers had a worse impact on survival, regardless of the number of cases (Fig. 8.7). In other words, while the optimal number of cases per center is still left to be understood, efforts should be made to centralize patients to networks of excellence, in order to prevent patients being treated at hospitals performing a median of 1/2 cases/year. For the future, efforts should be made to better identify the threshold of new cases per year above which there will be no further improvement of OS, in order to establish guidelines for patient referral also within the networks.

Besides volume, criteria for defining referral centers include multidisciplinarity, availability of facilities needed to properly apply clinical practice guidelines, prospective data collection, publication of outcomes, involvement in clinical and translational research, professional clinical and scientific education programs on the disease. The main medical societies have taken action in Europe and are presently lobbying the European Parliament as well as the governments of the different European countries to foster regionalization of sarcoma care.

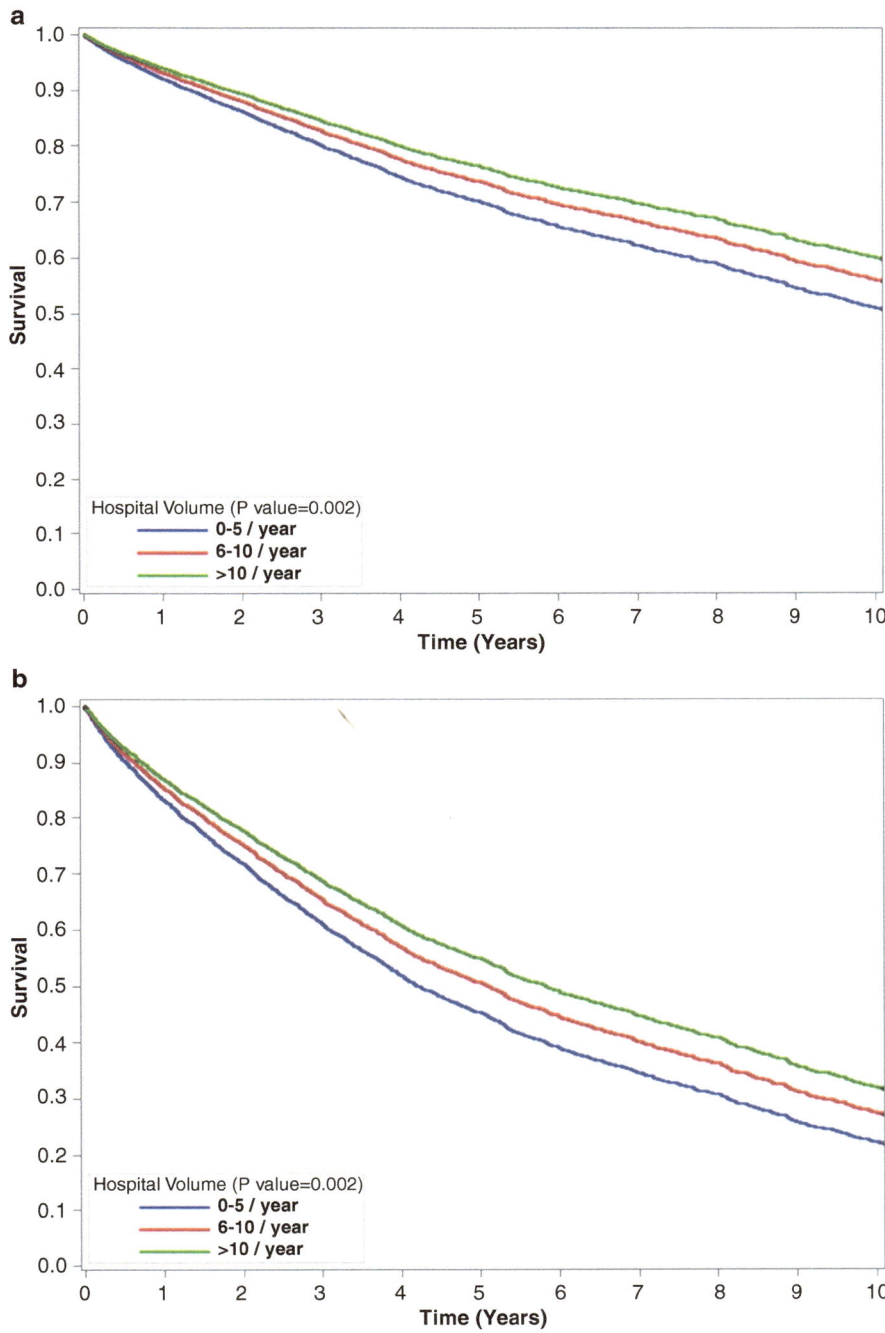

Fig. 8.5 Overall survival of patients affected by low-grade RPS (**a**) and by intermediate- or high-grade RPS (**b**) by center case volume: 0–5 (*blue line*), 6–10 (*red line*), and >10 (*green line*) primary new cases per year. *RPS* retroperitoneal sarcoma. (Reproduced with permission from [15])

Fig. 8.6 Hazard ratio of overall death (**a**) and 90-day mortality (**b**) stratified by annual surgical volume. (Reproduced with permission from [16])

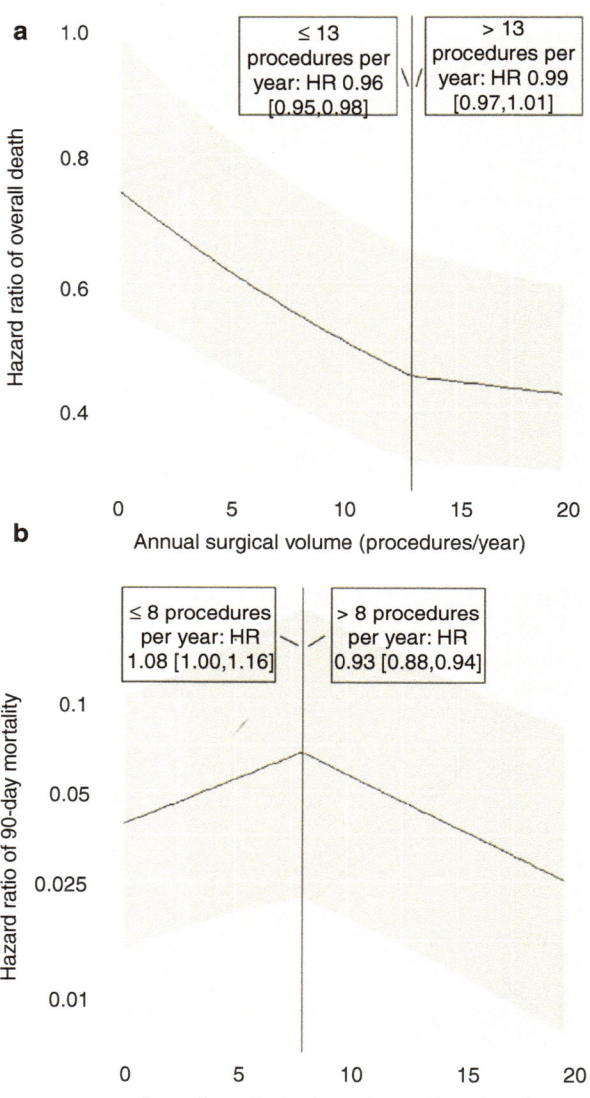

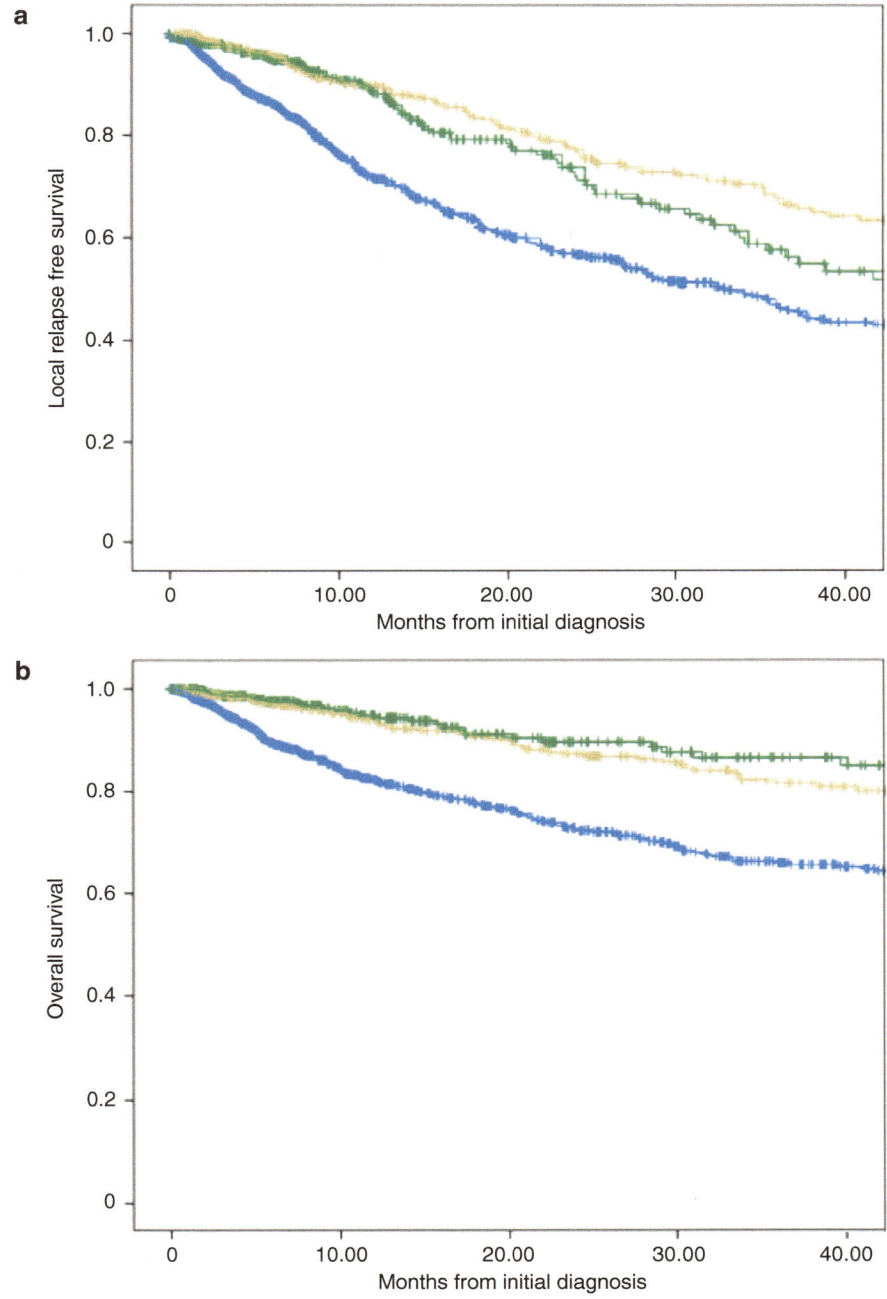

Fig. 8.7 Local relapse-free survival (**a**) and overall survival (**b**) of patients operated outside NETSARC centers (*blue line*) and within NETSARC centers operating <10 (*green line*) or >10 (*brown line*) new patients affected by primary soft tissue sarcoma originating at any site per year. (Reproduced with permission from [11])

8.5   Network of Excellence

Indeed, sarcoma are rare cancers. Five-year survival is lower for rare cancers than common cancers (49% vs. 63%) due to the biology of the diseases, adequacies of diagnosis and treatment, scarcity of effective therapies, and insufficient evidence-based treatment guidelines. In this context, it is necessary to invest on population-based registries to estimate incidence and survival and to define reference centers or collaborative networks with very specific expertise on rare malignancies, leading the way of diagnosis and treatment. In Europe, the surveillance of rare cancers in Europe, the RARECARE project, provided data from European population-based cancer registries to measure for the first time the burden of rare cancers in Europe. In addition, the project Information Network on Rare Cancers (RARECAREnet) was designed to gather epidemiological information on rare cancers, to allow for indicators and time trends at the country level, and to evaluate the level of centralization in Europe. In a recent report from RARECAREnet significant progress was reported for STS, consisting of a 3% increase in 5-year survival from 1999–2001 to 2007–2009, probably due to the recent trend toward centralization of sarcoma patients, who are more likely to benefit from a multidisciplinary approach in sarcoma comprehensive centers. To ensure appropriate, timely and high-quality care, a quality management system must be in place in each sarcoma center or network. The quality management system must ensure continuity of care for patients, the involvement in cancer care pathways, and the reporting of patient outcomes and experience. Periodic audits within the center/network or at a national level are necessary to review the past activity, discuss changes in protocols and procedures, and improve the performance of the unit/center. Among the European virtuous examples, we can find the National Institute of Health and Care Excellence (NICE) in England and Wales, and the abovementioned NETSARC. In detail, the NICE aims to ensure an appropriate multidisciplinary diagnostic and treatment pathway to sarcoma patients. France has clinical and pathology networks (NETSARC and RRePS) that provide patients with a systematic diagnosis and help to access treatment in specialized centers.

In Italy, the Italian Rare Cancers Network (RTR, Rete Tumori Rari), including 150 institutions, was established as a clinical collaborative effort to improve quality of care in adults with rare solid cancers. Moreover, it promotes collaborative clinical research by encouraging accrual into clinical trials and observational studies. In detail, clinical cases are shared within the RTR in order to rationalize access to distant referral centers and to minimize patient migration. A web resource is adopted to anonymously share the patients' data and images. A teleradiology resource is available, while a pathology review is arranged through transfer of paraffin-embedded specimens and upload of consultations. From 2000 to 2019, more than 10,000 cases of sarcoma have been uploaded. Every year 800 consultations are delivered and 1000 sarcoma cases are reviewed pathologically, with the diagnosis being changed in 33% of them.

8.6   Conclusions

In conclusion, the management of sarcomas is complex because of their biological diversity and the broad anatomical presentations. Specific expertise is required to improve outcomes and this mandates centralization in view of the rarity of the disease. Every effort should be made to foster the regionalization of sarcoma care and the implementation of networks to maximize the chance of cure. Besides the scientific data and guidelines provided by the scientific community, patient associations and regulators should take action to minimize disparities at a country and European level and to increase the rate of patients initially treated at sarcoma referral centers. This will have a major impact not only on the outcome of the single patient but also on the cost-benefit ratio for the health systems, with an obvious benefit also for payers and care providers worldwide.

References

1. Casali PG, Abecassis N, Bauer S, et al. Soft tissue and visceral sarcomas: ESMO–EURACAN clinical practice guidelines for diagnosis, treatment and follow-up. Ann Oncol. 2018;29(Suppl 4):iv51–67.
2. Gundle KR, Kafchinski L, Gupta S, et al. Analysis of margin classification systems for assessing the risk of local recurrence after soft tissue sarcoma resection. J Clin Oncol. 2018;36(7):704–9.
3. Gronchi A, Casali PG, Mariani L, et al. Status of surgical margins and prognosis in adult soft tissue sarcomas of the extremities: a series of patients treated at a single institution. J Clin Oncol. 2005;23(1):96–104.
4. Gronchi A, Lo Vullo S, Colombo C, et al. Extremity soft tissue sarcoma in a series of patients treated at a single institution. The local control directly impacts survival. Ann Surg. 2010;251(3):506–11.
5. Gronchi A, Verderio P, De Paoli A, et al. Quality of surgery and neoadjuvant combined therapy in the ISG-GEIS trial on soft tissue sarcomas of limbs and trunk wall. Ann Oncol. 2013;24(3):817–23.
6. Dingley B, Fiore M, Gronchi A. Personalizing surgical margins in retroperitoneal sarcomas: an update. Expert Rev Anticancer Ther. 2019;19(7):613–31.
7. Antritsch E, Beishon M, Bielack S, et al. ECCO essential requirements for quality cancer care: soft tissue sarcoma in adults and bone sarcoma. A critical review. Crit Rev Oncol Hematol. 2017;110:94–105.
8. Bonvalot S, Gronchi A, Le Pechoux C, et al. STRASS (EORTC 62092): a phase III randomized study of preoperative radiotherapy plus surgery versus surgery alone for patients with retroperitoneal sarcoma. J Clin Oncol. 2019;37(15 Suppl):11001. https://doi.org/10.1200/JCO.2019.37.15_suppl.11001.
9. Derbel O, Heudel PE, Cropet C, et al. Survival impact of centralization and clinical guidelines for soft tissue sarcoma (a prospective and exhaustive population-based cohort). PLoS One. 2017;12(2):e0158406. https://doi.org/10.1371/journal.pone.0158406.
10. Blay JY, Honoré C, Stoeckle E, et al. Surgery in reference centers improves survival of sarcoma patients: a nationwide study. Ann Oncol. 2019;30(7):1143–53.
11. Blay JY, Bonvalot S, Gouin F, et al. Criteria for reference centers for sarcomas: volume but also long-term multidisciplinary organisation. Ann Oncol. 2019;30(12):2008–9.
12. Kalaiselvan R, Malik AK, Rao R, et al. Impact of centralization of services on outcomes in a rare tumour: retroperitoneal sarcomas. Eur J Surg Oncol. 2019;45(2):249–53.

13. Bonvalot S, Gaignard E, Stoeckle E, et al. Survival benefit of the surgical management of retroperitoneal sarcoma in a reference center: a nationwide study of the French Sarcoma Group from the NetSarc database. Ann Surg Oncol. 2019;26(7):2286–93.
14. Villano AM, Zeymo A, McDermott J, et al. Regionalization of retroperitoneal sarcoma surgery to high-volume hospitals: missed opportunities for outcome improvement. J Oncol Pract. 2019;15(3):e247–61.
15. Keung EZ, Chiang YJ, Cormier JN, et al. Treatment at low-volume hospitals is associated with reduced short-term and long-term outcomes for patients with retroperitoneal sarcoma. Cancer. 2018;124(23):4495–503.
16. Villano AM, Zeymo A, Chan KS, et al. Identifying the minimum volume threshold for retroperitoneal soft tissue sarcoma resection: merging national data with consensus expert opinion. J Am Coll Surg. 2020;230(1):151–60.e2.
17. Raut CP, Bonvalot S, Gronchi A. A call to action: why sarcoma surgery needs to be centralized. Cancer. 2018;124(23):4452–4.

Volume-Outcome Relationship in Breast Surgery

9

Mario Taffurelli, Corrado Tinterri, Emilia Marrazzo, and Margherita Serra

9.1 Introduction

Breast cancer is the most common cancer amongst women in industrialized countries. In 2018 there were about 55,000 new cases in Italy alone, mainly in the North-Center areas of the country. The probability of developing sporadic breast cancer (about 95% of all cases) is estimated at 12% (1 in 8 women), whereas in the case of hereditary/familial tumors caused by the mutation of the acknowledged BRCA 1 and 2 genes the estimated probability is much higher, around 60%. The incidence of breast cancer is slightly increasing, while in the last decade there has been a decrease in mortality, estimated at around 0.4% per year. Today, breast cancer represents 29% of all cancers and is the most frequently diagnosed malignancy in women, accounting for 41% of cancers in women aged 0–49, 35% in those aged 50–69 years, and 21% in women older than 70 years. Moreover, it is the leading cause of death in women in all age groups: 29% of deaths between 0 and 49 years, 23% between 50 and 69 years and 16% among women over 70 years old. There are differences between macro-areas with a higher incidence in the North (123.4 cases per 100,000 inhabitants) compared with Center (103.8 cases per 100,000 inhabitants) and the South and Islands (93.1 cases per 100,000 inhabitants), probably due to differences in access to mammography screening and to heterogeneity in the distribution of risk factors for malignant breast cancer (early menses, late menopause, absence of pregnancies and breastfeeding, use of hormone replacement therapy in menopause, diet, physical activity, smoking, alcohol consumption).

M. Taffurelli (✉) · M. Serra
Breast Unit, Department of Woman, Child and Urological Diseases,
Policlinico Sant'Orsola-Malpighi, University of Bologna, Bologna, Italy
e-mail: mario.taffurelli@aosp.bo.it; margherita.serra@aosp.bo.it

C. Tinterri · E. Marrazzo
Breast Unit, Humanitas Clinical and Research Center IRCCS, Rozzano, Milan, Italy
e-mail: corrado.tinterri@cancercenter.humanitas.it; emilia.marrazzo@humanitas.it

© Springer Nature Switzerland AG 2021
M. Montorsi (ed.), *Volume-Outcome Relationship in Oncological Surgery*,
Updates in Surgery, https://doi.org/10.1007/978-3-030-51806-6_9

9.2   Treatment of Breast Cancer: Endpoints and Outcomes

Mortality reduction is no doubt associated with an adequate diagnosis, treatment and follow-up, which can only be achieved through a correct diagnostic-therapeutic care pathway, possible within a *breast unit*, in which the management of the disease is based on the principle of multidisciplinarity.

In 2014, the Italian Permanent Conference for Relations between the State, the Regions and the Autonomous Provinces of Trento and Bolzano approved a document of the Ministry of Health, setting out the criteria that such breast units had to meet [1]. These criteria are mainly based on the requirements already established by the European Society of Breast Cancer Specialists (EUSOMA), the most important European scientific society on breast cancer [2].

The EUSOMA requirements, in addition to the volume of cases treated, state that all cases should be discussed jointly by a multidisciplinary team that must include a radiologist, pathologist, surgeon, oncological radiotherapist, medical oncologist, and case-manager nurse, giving the care pathway multidisciplinary and multiprofessional significance (*core team*). In addition, these specialists should be dedicated to breast pathology, diagnostics and treatment, establishing for each a specific working time. This is because, while indispensable, the volume of cases treated is not sufficient; in fact, dedication to the pathology expands not only knowledge about one's own discipline, but also about the others included in the core team, thus making it possible to decide on the most adequate diagnostic-therapeutic process for achieving a good final outcome. Other professionals must be occasionally added to the core team depending on the single case, such as plastic surgeons, nuclear radiologists, physical therapists and physiotherapists, psycho-oncologists, geneticists, gynecologists and experts in fertility preservation. By treating breast cancer in such a multidisciplinary and multiprofessional setting, an improvement of about 18% in overall survival could be achieved [3].

The volume of cases treated is directly proportional to the results obtained regarding both survival, as the primary endpoint, and quality of life of the patient. We refer in particular to the aesthetic result than can be achieved by a surgical team dedicated to conservative breast surgery, with the possibility to perform mastectomies followed by immediate breast reconstruction, to utilize the most modern techniques which preserve the skin mantle and based on current guidelines, the nipple (skin- and/or nipple-sparing mastectomies) and to reduce the number of reinterventions for positive margins following conservative treatment, which obviously can have an extremely negative psychological impact on the patient, as well as significantly increasing the cost of care (two admissions = two procedures).

The literature is rich in contributions that show how the volume of cases is directly correlated to the primary endpoint, which, as in any oncological pathology, is survival.

A recent survey [4] that used the American College of Surgeons Database on 1,602,051 women treated surgically for breast cancer in the US, showed clearly how the volume of cases treated is directly correlated to survival. The examined sample was divided into patients treated at low-volume centers with less than 148 cases/

year, intermediate-volume centers with between 149 and 298 cases/year and high-volume centers with more than 298 cases/year. There were a total of 1277 hospitals that treated breast cancer, of which 1044 were low-volume, 181 intermediate and 52 high-volume centers, with a mean number of cases treated per year of 52,194 and 385, respectively. The univariate analysis showed a significantly higher overall survival in patients treated at a high-volume center rather than an intermediate- or a low-volume one at 5- and 10-year follow-up (91% vs. 90% vs. 87% at 5 years; 77% vs. 75% vs. 70% at 10 years). Multivariate analysis confirmed the survival benefit in high-volume centers with an 11% advantage over low-volume centers. It is interesting to note that the greatest benefit was found among patients treated for ductal carcinoma in situ, which are notoriously the ones that require a more complex treatment, from both a technical and a decisional point of view, in which the experience of a multidisciplinary team has a fundamental role.

Previous studies with smaller samples [5] stated that the relation between higher volume and better outcome was associated with the high level of clinical competence of all specialists involved and above all with their ability to manage adjuvant treatments (chemotherapy, hormonal therapy, and radiotherapy), a less frequent practice in the low-volume centers. In a series published in the *Annals of Surgery* [4], the treatment pathway taken, as in adjuvant or neo-adjuvant therapy, showed no impact on survival, while the volume of cases treated, at a level of both facility and number of procedures, was an independent and decisive factor.

Scientific evidence to date has not identified precise minimum or maximum volume thresholds, but it is possible to establish an interval, below which the risk of worse outcome is increased. As established at a European level, only centers that treat at least 150 cases per year can be defined as "breast units". Although the performance of 150 interventions per year has been recognized as the minimum necessary volume, there is still no agreement on the minimal volume per surgeon. As previously mentioned, EUSOMA has proposed as a threshold 50 breast cancer operations per year, while for the French National Institute of Cancer it should be 30 procedures.

In a review published in the *European Journal of Surgical Oncology* in 2010 [6], it emerged from several studies that the relation between volume and outcome was dependent on the age and comorbidities of the patient; in an increasingly ageing population, often with other concomitant conditions, reduced autonomy and under important pharmacological therapies, treating elderly patients in low-volume centers, which are not equipped with specific treatment services (physical therapy, pain therapy, nutritional therapy, etc.) or intensive care units, was associated with an increase in morbidity and mortality due to short- and long-term complications, not seen in larger centers that provide such services.

The relation between volume and outcome in terms of survival would depend on the experience, standardization and homogeneity of the treatment offered by high-volume centers, thus emphasizing the need to centralize breast cancer cases, regardless of age and comorbidities, in order to provide a survival advantage at any age or clinical condition.

In 2012 the Emilia-Romagna Region carried out a study on around 6000 cases of operated patients, who showed a statistically higher survival when treated in dedicated centers with at least 150 interventions per year. The survival curves showed a significantly lower delta in patients treated in centers performing less than 50 interventions per year.

The volume of activity not only has an impact on survival—and therefore the long-term expectations of the patients—but it is also decisive in the short-term, specifically for the need for reintervention. Despite the fact that in dedicated centers conservative surgery is more common than in low-volume ones, where destructive surgery is performed more often, there is an inversely proportional relation between volume of activity and the risk of reintervention because of positive margins. This aspect has been widely analyzed in the literature. In 2013 McDermott et al. carried out a study to evaluate the correlation between volume of activity per surgeon and performance indicators, such as the rate of conservative versus destructive interventions, sentinel lymph node biopsy versus radical axillary lymph node dissection in patients with no clinical evidence of axillary involvement (cN0) and reinterventions for positive margins. The analysis of more than 80,000 cases showed that in dedicated high-volume centers (defined as more than 50 interventions per year) there was a significant difference in the number of conservative interventions, reinterventions and sentinel lymph node biopsies compared to centers with lower volumes. However, the authors concluded that such an advantage was not directly dependent on the single operator ability, but it was due to the role of the multidisciplinary discussion in the patient management. The early diagnosis by dedicated radiologists, the availability of highly specialized infrastructure, such as nuclear medicine, and dedicated pathologists, it was possible to perform more sentinel lymph node biopsies than immediate axillary lymph node dissections, conservative rather than destructive surgery and to avoid reintervention, as each case had been accurately studied preoperatively by a panel of experts [7].

In the surgical treatment of breast cancer, the aesthetic result is important and, if unsatisfactory, it may have a negative psychological effect on the patients. Using plastic surgery techniques is now essential in breast surgery to avoid or minimize the aesthetic impact after the partial removal of the gland, while maintaining oncologic radicality.

Oncoplastic surgery prevents breast deformities and is based on the integration of plastic surgery techniques for immediate reshaping after wide excision for breast cancer. There are two levels of oncoplastic surgery based on excision volume and the complexity of the reshaping technique. Level I is indicated for resections less than 20% of the breast volume and allows easy reshaping of the breast. Level II is for larger resections and a mammoplasty technique is required. A level I approach is based on recentralization of the nipple-areola complex, no skin excision is required, and the resulting glandular defect can usually be filled by advancement of adjacent tissue. Level II techniques are based on different mammoplasty techniques and allow greater volume resections, they involve extensive skin excision and breast reshaping. They result in a significantly smaller, rounder breast. The procedures are superior pedicle mammoplasty, inferior pedicle mammoplasty, round block mammoplasty, inverted T or vertical-scar mammoplasty with nipple-areola complex resection. Surgeons have to identify and choose the appropriate oncoplastic technique, based on excision volume, tumor location, and glandular density. This is only possible in dedicated centers, with a high volume of patients. By contrast, when a destructive intervention is required, reconstruction options through tissue expanders or implants or autologous tissue (pedunculated or free) when indicated, must be offered, and two surgical teams are required (plastic and general surgeons), with particular experience in microsurgery. These reconstructions require precise surgical indications (deep inferior epigastric perforator or free flap), and they have to be centralized into high-volume hospitals. The collaboration between oncologic and plastic surgeons, possible in high-volume centers, guarantees the use of the best and most up-to-date reconstruction techniques.

9.3   The Current Italian Situation

Analyzing the Italian data provided by the National Agency for Health Services (AGENAS, Agenzia Nazionale per i Servizi Sanitari) there is an improvement in breast reconstruction techniques. In fact, the proportion of reconstruction interventions occurring during the same destructive intervention went from 35.5% in 2010 to 50% in 2017, and even higher in 2018; the Italian average is 50% (https://www. agenas.gov.it).

Despite the lack of studies evaluating the relation between the volume of cases and aesthetic results, an indirect assessment can be made by analyzing the rate of surgical complications (hemorrhage, infection, dehiscence) which is significantly lower in high-volume centers [8].

A survey published in 2016 [9] showed that, in a sample of 300 patients with primary breast cancer treated by conservative surgery, the most common and most dissatisfying problem was the dislocation of the nipple-areola complex, which is caused by a deficiency of skin and gland. The deformity appears much more evident in smaller breasts, in which the portion of the glandular tissue removed is greater than in breasts with medium or bigger volume. Thus, the preoperative multidisciplinary assessment, including the contribution of an expert plastic surgeon, is essential for a correct therapeutic strategy and a good aesthetic outcome [10]. Another study published in 2013 proved that patients treated in multidisciplinary centers and provided with detailed information about the expectations after surgery showed greater satisfaction about the final aesthetic result [11].

In Italy, the collaboration between health facilities, health professionals and the Ministry of Health has made it possible to implement a National Outcome Evaluation Program (PNE, Programma Nazionale Esiti), developed by AGENAS. The PNE provides, at national level, comparative assessments of efficacy, safety, efficiency and quality of care produced within the health service. The indicators are discussed within the PNE Committee, composed of representatives of the Ministry of Health, Regions, Autonomous Provinces, and scientific institutions. The use of indicators for assessing the quality of oncology care must be considered an essential element to verify the effective capacity of the system to better assist cancer patients and to re-orient and, if necessary, correct the dysfunctions detected in terms of professional skills, organization of services and their interconnections and interrelations (networks), development and innovation. The PNE is used to measure the quality of care provided in the various Italian hospitals and to analyze equity of access to adequate cancer care (volumes and mortality) and to some oncological surgeries (surgery for breast cancer and pancreas) by area of residence (commissioning function). In addition to being an indicator of the quality of assistance, activity volumes can be used to verify the structure and distribution of the hospital care offer and to guide the reorganization of care networks, including oncological networks.

The decision as to which volume threshold to use as a reference must be based on criteria that depend on the context and sustainability of the results deriving from these choices. An excessive fragmentation of activities reduces the quality of care outcomes and causes a possible waste of resources, while an excessive concentration leads to the hypertrophy of few facilities, with negative consequences on the accessibility of services, possible diseconomies of scale and marginal benefits in terms of quality assistance.

The PNE contains about 170 outcome indicators, of which 34 belong to the oncology area and are focused on surgical procedures and activity volumes and, at regional or provincial level, further reference thresholds have been proposed for a greater number of oncological conditions.

In the light of this qualitative reference in healthcare, the Ministry of Health's Decree of April 2, 2015, defining "the qualitative, structural, technological and quantitative standards for hospital care" [12], highlighted the relationship observed between volumes of activity, treatment outcomes and specific number of facilities for each value; this makes it possible to carry out impact assessments for the choice of volume thresholds and outcome thresholds.

The identified thresholds apply to all public and private accredited entities. In the meanings of these definitions, also of a qualitative nature, taking into account also the aspects related to the efficiency in the use of the facilities, the following minimum thresholds of volume of activity are defined as valid in breast surgery: 150 annual interventions on breast cancer cases for a complex facility.

In the various hospital structures it is therefore indispensable to provide network training mechanisms that enhance the learning opportunities and the acquisition of the competences present in the various nodes of the system, so as to avoid a progressive impoverishment of the professionals who work in the operating units that attend a series of lesser complexity.

The impact of the work of both the PNE, AGENAS and the scientific community that in Italy revolves around the issue of breast cancer (Associazione Senonetwork Italia, www.senonetwork.it) has changed the healthcare offer for this pathology. The data collected in an investigation of a Commission of the Italian Senate on various diseases, including breast cancer, published in 2011, photographed a reality of Italian hospitals in which the percentage of cases treated in centers with volumes greater than 150 was 12% [13]. The data currently published by AGENAS relating to the treatment of breast cancer in Italian health facilities in 2017 showed a percentage of over 70% of cases treated in centers with volumes greater than 135 cases (https://pne.agenas.it).

Central to the awareness of the population and the attention of women with breast cancer to addressing dedicated facilities has been the constant and wide-spread work of the women's associations, in particular Europa Donna, a social promotion association whose objective is to effectively respond to needs and rights of women with breast cancer, presenting themselves as the main movement of opinion on the subject.

Continuing to analyze the PNE/AGENAS data (https://pne.agenas.it), the proportion of new resection interventions within 120 days of conservative intervention for malignant breast cancer has improved over time, going from 12.3% in 2010 to 7.4% in 2017 and decreasing even in the last year of measurement. Analyzing the specific Region by Region data for 2017 reported by AGENAS, there is an increase in admissions to dedicated facilities in the same region (Table 9.1), thanks to breast units that on a local voluntary basis have developed a specific and multidisciplinary breast care offer.

It is therefore necessary both in terms of increased survival and in terms of reintervention and aesthetic results to centralize patients suffering from breast cancer to high-volume centers, where they can be treated by multidisciplinary and dedicated team.

Table 9.1 Admissions of patients of Italian Regions for breast cancer surgery (year 2017)

| | | Of which in structures of | |
| | | The same Region | Other Regions |
Region (or autonomous province)	Total admissions	(%)	(%)
Piedmont	4323	87.4	12.6
Valle d'Aosta	118	92.5	7.5
Liguria	1528	82.2	17.8
Lombardy	14,545	98.9	1.1
Bolzano	465	94.6	5.4
Trento	492	88.7	11.3
Veneto	5257	93.1	6.9
Friuli Venezia Giulia	1974	97.7	2.3
Emilia-Romagna	5400	92.4	7.6
Marche	1683	86.0	14.0
Tuscany	4170	94.0	6.0
Umbria	1069	88.4	11.6
Lazio	6218	95.3	4.7
Abruzzo	1194	86.5	13.5
Molise	210	88.5	11.5
Campania	3920	88.4	11.6
Puglia	2926	85.0	15.0
Basilicata	402	70.6	29.4
Calabria	820	55.2	44.8
Sicily	3569	87.9	12.1
Sardinia	1396	83.5	16.5

Data from: AGENAS—Programma Nazionale Esiti (https://pne.agenas.it)

References

1. Intesa, ai sensi dell'articolo 8, comma 6 della legge 5 giugno 2003, n. 131, sul documento recante "Linee di indirizzo sulle modalità organizzative ed assistenziali della rete dei Centri di Senologia". Conferenza permanente per i rapporti tra lo Stato, le Regioni e le Province Autonome di Trento e Bolzano, 18 dicembre 2014 [Agreement, pursuant to article 8, paragraph 6, of the law of June 5, 2003, n. 131, concerning the "Guidelines on the organizational and care methods of the network of Senology Centers" Permanent Conference for Relations between the State, the Regions and the Autonomous Provinces of Trento and Bolzano, December 18, 2014]. http://archivio.statoregioni.it/Documenti/DOC_045999_185%20%20 CSR%20PUNTO%204.pdf.
2. Biganzoli L, Marotti L, Hart CD, et al. Quality indicators in breast cancer care: An update from the EUSOMA working group. Eur J Cancer. 2017;86:59–81.
3. Kesson EM, Allardice GM, George WD, et al. Effects of multidisciplinary team working on breast cancer survival: retrospective, comparative, interventional cohort study of 13,722 women. BMJ. 2012;344:e2718. https://doi.org/10.1136/bmj.e2718.
4. Greenup RA, Obeng-Gyasi S, Thomas S, et al. The effect of hospital volume on breast cancer mortality. Ann Surg. 2018;267(2):375–81.
5. Kong AL, Pezzin LE, Nattinger AB. Identifying patterns of breast cancer care provided at high-volume hospitals: a classification and regression tree analysis. Breast Cancer Res Treat. 2015;153(3):689–98.
6. Gooiker GA, van Gijn W, Post PN, et al. A systematic review and meta-analysis of the volume-outcome relationship in the surgical treatment of breast cancer. Are breast cancer patients better of with a high-volume provider? Eur J Surg Oncol. 2010;36(Suppl 1):S27–35.
7. McDermott AM, Wall DM, Waters PS, et al. Surgeon and breast unit volume-outcome relationships in breast cancer surgery and treatment. Ann Surg. 2013;258(5):808–13; discussion 813–4.
8. Guller U, Safford S, Pietrobon R, et al. High hospital volume is associated with better outcomes for breast cancer surgery: analysis of 233,247 patients. World J Surg. 2005;29(8):994–9; discussion 999–1000.
9. Dahlbäck C, Manjer J, Rehn M, et al. Determinants for patient satisfaction regarding aesthetic outcome and skin sensitivity after breast-conserving surgery. World J Surg Oncol. 2016;14(1):303. https://doi.org/10.1186/s12957-016-1053-8.
10. Chen K, Feng CJ, Ma H, et al. Preoperative breast volume evaluation of one-stage immediate breast reconstruction using three-dimensional surface imaging and a printed mold. J Chin Med Assoc. 2019;82(9):732–9.
11. Ho AL, Klassen AF, Cano S, et al. Optimizing patient-centered care in breast reconstruction: the importance of preoperative information and patient-physician communication. Plast Reconstr Surg. 2013;132(2):212e–20e.
12. Decreto Ministeriale 2 aprile 2015 n. 70. Regolamento recante definizione degli standard qualitativi, strutturali, tecnologici e quantitativi relativi all'assistenza ospedaliera [Ministerial Decree April 2, 2015, n. 70. "Regulation on the definition of quality, structural, technological and quantitative standards relating to hospital care"]. https://www.camera.it/ temiap/2016/09/23/OCD177-2353.pdf.
13. Atti dell'Indagine conoscitiva svolta dalla XII Commissione permanente del Senato (Igiene e Sanità) n. 36, luglio 2011, XVI legislatura "Malattie ad andamento degenerativo di particolare rilevanza sociale, con specifico riguardo al tumore della mammella, alle malattie reumatiche croniche ed alla sindrome HIV" [Proceedings of the fact-finding survey carried out by the XII Permanent Commission of the Senate (Hygiene and Health) n. 36, July 2011, Legislature XVI "Degenerative diseases of particular social significance, with specific regard to breast cancer, chronic rheumatic diseases, and HIV syndrome"]. https://www.senato.it/application/ xmanager/projects/senato/file/indagine_conoscitiva_n.36.pdf.

Volume-Outcome Relationship in Endocrine Surgery

10

Rocco Bellantone, Francesco Pennestrì, Carmela De Crea, Celestino Pio Lombardi, Mario Testini, Giorgio De Toma, and Marco Raffaelli

10.1 Introduction

Forty years ago, Luft et al. [1, 2] examined the relationship between volume and outcomes in surgery and questioned whether surgical care should be regionalized to optimize outcomes. Looking at 12 different procedures of varying complexity at 1498 hospitals, they found major differences in selected procedures. Indeed, in specific surgical operations, mortality rates were significantly lower in high-volume centers, while others showed no association between hospital volume and outcomes. These data sparked significant interest, and numerous studies have evaluated this phenomenon over the last four decades. Many studies show that patient mortality decreases and patient outcomes improve when complex operations are performed at high-volume centers [1–5]. This is true for many surgical procedures, and there is no doubt that it is related to multiple factors, including several independent of the surgeon [3–5]. This is exemplified by high-risk surgeries requiring a complex perioperative management, for instance surgical treatment of pancreas, lung, esophagus, or colon cancers. High-volume centers tend to be larger and likely have advanced resources, which include an array of specialists, advanced intensive care units, specialized surgical and anesthesia teams, sophisticated blood banks, and the

R. Bellantone · F. Pennestrì · C. De Crea (✉) · C. P. Lombardi · M. Raffaelli
Centro Dipartimentale di Chirurgia Endocrina e dell'Obesità, Fondazione Policlinico Universitario Agostino Gemelli IRCCS, Università Cattolica del Sacro Cuore, Rome, Italy
e-mail: rocco.bellantone@unicatt.it; francesco.pennestri@policlinicogemelli.it; carmela.decrea@unicatt.it; celestinopio.lombardi@unicatt.it; marco.raffaelli@unicatt.it

M. Testini
U.O.C. Chirurgia Generale Universitaria V. Bonomo, Università degli Studi di Bari Aldo Moro, A.O.U. Consorziale Policlinico di Bari, Bari, Italy
e-mail: mario.testini@uniba.it

G. De Toma
Dipartimento di Chirurgia P. Valdoni, Sapienza University of Rome, Rome, Italy
e-mail: giorgio.detoma@uniroma1.it

© Springer Nature Switzerland AG 2021
M. Montorsi (ed.), *Volume-Outcome Relationship in Oncological Surgery*, Updates in Surgery, https://doi.org/10.1007/978-3-030-51806-6_10

capacity to accommodate the most complex comorbid conditions [5–7]. More commonly performed procedures requiring a less complex perioperative management, including vagotomy and cholecystectomy, did not show a relationship between hospital volume and patient outcomes [2].

However, several studies have shown that morbidity and mortality are decreased when the surgical providers have high operative volumes, regardless of the volume of the center [6, 8, 9]. While intuitively logical, it has only recently been shown that increased surgical volume improves outcomes [6, 8, 9]. This has contributed to surgical subspecialization, with the expectation that surgeons performing fewer types of procedures at higher volumes develop advanced techniques, improved judgment, and, therefore, enhanced outcomes. Within endocrine surgery, a subspecialty of general surgery, thyroidectomy, parathyroidectomy, and adrenalectomy are cited as procedures where surgeon experience appears to affect outcomes [10–14].

In the present chapter, we will summarize the literature about the correlation between surgical outcomes and volumes of centers and surgeons, in endocrine surgery. It is important to specify that, considering the rarity of the endocrine oncological disease, mainly with regard to adrenal, parathyroid and gastroenteropancreatic tumors, the reported clinical series are very limited and heterogeneous and the existing literature mostly refers to benign disease. As thyroid cancers have a higher incidence, some of the mentioned studies will comprise several reports specifically dealing with volumes and outcomes in thyroid carcinomas.

10.2   Thyroid Surgery

A number of studies published over the past 20 years have shown that thyroid surgery-specific complications (i.e., hypocalcemia, recurrent laryngeal nerve palsy, and postoperative hematoma) as well as length of stay and general postoperative complications are improved with increasing surgeon caseload [15–23]. However, although the relationship between surgeon volume and outcome is established, there is no accepted threshold to define a 'high-volume' surgeon, nor a method to determine its value [9]. Consequently, the volume-outcome thyroid studies each have different definitions of high-volume surgery [11].

Furthermore, in various countries, including Switzerland and Austria, numerous thyroid surgeries are performed in hospitals with a low annual number of operations: in 2016, 48.6% of the hospitals providing thyroid surgery performed between 1 and 30 thyroidectomies [12]. To provide the same perioperative management standards in all hospitals, and to maintain lower complication rates in thyroid surgery, different consensus guidelines have been written by independent professional scientific organizations worldwide [14, 24–31].

For instance, in 1998 Sosa et al. [15] published a statewide cross-sectional analysis including 5860 patients. Individual surgeons were categorized according to the total 6-year volume (1–9, 10–29, 30–100, and >100 thyroidectomies). Similarly, total hospital volume was grouped in four categories (1–99, 100–199, 200–300, >300). Results showed that the highest-volume surgeons had the shortest length of stay and the lowest complication rate, while hospital volume had no consistent association with outcomes.

However, these results were refuted in 2000, when Thomusch et al. [32] reported a prospective multicentric study including 7266 patients who underwent thyroid resection for benign diseases over a 1-year period (1998). Surgeons were now categorized according to their experience (trainee vs. specialist), while hospitals were categorized as low-, intermediate- and high-volume (<50, 50–150 and >150 procedures, respectively). Initially, no significant difference was found among hospital groups regarding post-thyroidectomy morbidity and mortality rates. In the logistic regression analyses for transient and permanent hypoparathyroidism, though, extent of resection (RR 1.5–1.8), recurrent goiter (RR 1.8–1.9), Graves' disease (RR 2.8), operative volumes of hospitals (RR 0.8–1.5), and patient gender (RR 2.1–2.3) were significant risk factors.

Furthermore, in 2008 Mitchell et al. [33] published a single-institution retrospective analysis on 335 thyroid and parathyroid reoperations. This time it was proved that many thyroid and parathyroid reoperations were avoidable, and that the majority of them were needed after the first surgery had been performed at low-volume centers [33]. Thus, in addition to decreased complication rates, thyroid and parathyroid surgery performed at high-volume centers would reduce the indication to reoperative surgery for inadequate initial surgical resection.

Studying again the relation with both surgical and center volumes, in 2010 Gourin et al. [17] reported a statewide cross-sectional analysis including 21,270 patients; individual surgeons were categorized according to the annual volume in low-, intermediate- and high-volume ($\leq$3, 4–24, >24 thyroidectomies/year). Similarly, hospital volume was divided into three categories ($\leq$22, 23–100, >100). Multiple logistic regression analyses of variables associated with thyroid surgery-specific complications revealed no association with hospital volume. On the contrary, an association with surgeon volume was shown, since high-volume surgeons had a lower incidence of laryngeal nerve injury (OR 0.46, $p < 0.01$) and hypocalcemia (OR 0.49, $p < 0.01$), coherently with the first studies.

Another fascinating insight was given by Duclos et al. [34] in 2012, when they reported a prospective cross-sectional multicentric study from five academic French hospitals, which included 28 surgeons and 3574 thyroid procedures. This time, the study showed that a 20-year practice was associated with an increased probability of both recurrent laryngeal nerve palsy (OR 3.06, CI 1.07–8.80, $p = 0.04$) and permanent hypoparathyroidism (OR 7.56, CI 1.79–31.99), $p = 0.01$). Interestingly, it was shown that surgeons' performance has a concave association with their length of experience ($p = 0.036$) and age ($p = 0.035$); surgeons aged 35–50 years had better outcomes than their younger and older colleagues did.

In 2013 Loyo et al. [19] released a nationwide cross-sectional analysis (Nationwide Inpatient Sample) including 871,644 patients. Individual surgeons were categorized according to their annual volume into very low-, low-, intermediate-, and high-volume ($\leq$3, 4–9, 9–23 and >24 thyroidectomies/year). Similarly, hospital volume was categorized into four categories ($\leq$25, 26–42, 43–76 and >76). Multiple logistic regression analysis of variables associated with thyroid surgery-specific complications demonstrated that recurrent laryngeal nerve palsy and hypocalcemia were significantly less likely for high-volume surgeons (OR 0.71, CI 0.53–0.95, p = 0.24 and OR 0.7, CI 0.57–0.88, p = 0.002, respectively). Once again, after having adjusted for surgeon volume, hospital volume was not associated with complication rate.

In 2013 González-Sánchez et al. [35] published a single-institution prospective cohort study including 225 patients and 8 surgeons (two endocrine surgery specialists with a caseload >40 procedures/year, and 6 non-endocrine specialized general surgeons with a caseload <5 procedures/year). This time, with surgeons categorized based on their specialization, it was shown that permanent recurrent laryngeal nerve palsy and hypocalcemia were significantly reduced for specialized high-volume surgeons (1/325 vs. 2/46, p = 0.04, and 3/130 vs. 3/16, p = 0.028, respectively).

Again, in 2013, Kandil et al. [18] reported a nationwide cross-sectional analysis (Health Care Utilization Project National Inpatient Sample [HCUP-NIS] data sets) including 46,261 patients. Individual surgeons were once again categorized according to the volume of procedures performed over the 10-year study period (low-, intermediate- and high-volume: <10, 10–99, ≥100 procedures, respectively). High-volume hospitals were instead defined as those above the 75th percentile regarding yearly caseload. Yet another time, it was proved that high-volume surgeons had a significantly lower rate of complications, while hospital volume had an inconsistent and marginal protective effect on postoperative outcomes.

Subsequently, in 2016, Al-Qurayshi et al. [36] presented a nationwide cross-sectional analysis using the National Inpatient Sample data-sets, including 77,863 patients. Surgeons were categorized based on their annual caseload (low-, intermediate- and high-volume: 1–3, 4–29, ≥30 thyroidectomies/year, respectively). Consistently with the previously quoted results, procedures performed by low-volume surgeons were associated with a higher risk of postoperative complications compared with those performed by high-volume surgeons (15.8% vs. 7.7%, OR 1.55, CI 1.19–2.03, p = 0.01).

One could thus conclude that surgeon's expertise (measured by surgical volume of procedures per year) is associated with favorable clinical as well as financial outcomes.

A further analysis was provided by Meltzer et al. [37], in 2016: they reported on a nationwide cohort study including 4909 patients who underwent total thyroidectomy between 2008 and 2013. Propensity-score matching was used for patients of low- (<20 thyroidectomies per year) and high-volume surgeons (>40 thyroidectomies per year). Results showed that high-volume surgeons had shorter operative times (2.4 vs. 3.0 h, $p < 0.05$), shorter lengths of stay (29.9 vs. 39.8 h, $p < 0.05$), and lower rate of all surgery-related complications (5.7% vs. 7.5%, $p < 0.05$), 30-day rates of hypocalcemia (4.9% vs. 7.0%, $p < 0.05$), and surgical site infection (0.3% vs. 1.0%, $p < 0.05$).

Liang et al. [38], in 2016, reported a nationwide cross-sectional analysis of data of 125,037 patients obtained by the Taiwan Bureau of National Health Insurance and systematic review and metanalysis of the literature. Surgeons were categorized into low- and high-volume (1–70 and >70 thyroidectomies/year, respectively), and hospitals were classified accordingly (1–200 and >200 thyroidectomies/year, respectively). The results showed that patients who underwent thyroidectomies performed by high-volume hospitals and surgeons had shorter length of stay and lower costs compared with those treated by low-volume hospitals and surgeons, coherently with the previously quoted study.

In 2016, Youngwirth et al. [39] proved an additional point by publishing an analysis of 31,129 patients with papillary thyroid cancer who had undergone total thyroidectomy obtained by querying the National Cancer Data Base (patients operated upon during the 1998–2006 period). The objective of the study was to determine the role of positive margins on these patients' survival. Patients were divided into three groups based on margin status (negative, microscopically positive, and macroscopically positive), and then a Cox proportional hazards model was developed to identify factors associated with survival. Of the 31,129 patients enrolled, 91.3% had negative margins, 8.1% had microscopically positive margins, and 0.6% had macroscopically positive margins. After multivariable adjustment, the findings showed that increasing patient age (OR 1.02, $p < 0.01$), government insurance (OR 1.20, $p < 0.01$), and no insurance (OR 1.34, $p = 0.01$) were associated with positive margins and thus with a compromised survival. Instead, this time reception of surgery at a high-volume facility (OR 0.72, $p < 0.01$) was protective; in conclusion, it was even shown that high-risk thyroid cancer patients should be referred to high-volume centers to optimize outcomes.

In 2017 Adam et al. [23] presented a nationwide cross-sectional analysis (Health Care Utilization Project-National Inpatient Sample [HCUP-NIS] data-sets) including 16,954 patients. Surgeons were categorized into low-volume ($\leq$25 procedures/ year) and high-volume (>25 procedures/year). Yet another time, patients undergoing thyroidectomy were more likely to have any complications (OR 1.52, CI 1.16–1.97, $p = 0.002$) and a longer hospital stay (+12%, $p = 0.006$) when the operation was performed by a low-volume surgeon.

Likewise, the nationwide cross-sectional analysis published in 2017 by Nouraei et al. [22] showed the superiority of high-volume surgeons: by using record of 72,594 patients obtained from the Hospital Episode Statistics (HES) data-set, the authors demonstrated that high-volume surgeons achieve lower complication rates, including lower vocal palsy rates, and length of stay.

Another nationwide cross-sectional analysis was published in 2019 by Aspinall et al. [11], who used records of 25,038 patients obtained from the United Kingdom Registry of Endocrine and Thyroid Surgery (UKRETS). In their study, age, retrosternal goiter, routine laryngoscopy, re-operation, nodal dissection, bilateral thyroidectomy, recurrent laryngeal nerve monitoring, and surgeon volume were significantly associated with recurrent laryngeal nerve palsy. Instead, postoperative hematoma showed no significant correlation to surgeon volume. However, categorization of annual rates showed that permanent hypoparathyroidism and recurrent laryngeal nerve palsy rates declined in surgeons performing >50 cases/year to a minimum of 3% and 2.6% respectively, in the highest volume annual rate group (>100 cases/ year). Once again, the authors concluded that surgeon annual operative volume is a factor in determining outcomes in thyroid surgery.

Finally, very interesting is the multicenter electronic survey published in 2019 by Jakob et al. [12], who investigated how the departments' annual number of thyroid surgeries correlates with adherence to consensus guidelines and implementation of measures for quality assurance. Patient management corresponded to the summarized recommendations in 64.0% of cases. Also intriguing is that adherence to the recommendations and implementation of measures for quality assurance were significantly more likely to occur with increasing numbers of surgeries performed ($p = 0.049$ and $p < 0.001$), all consistent with the majority of studies on this topic. Ninety-two departments provided thyroid cancer surgery, whereas 12/92 (13.0%) were not able to perform central and/or lateral neck dissection. The authors concluded that, while consensus guidelines are insufficiently implemented in thyroid surgery, quality management is associated with surgical volume.

10.3 Parathyroid Surgery

Since the 1980s, when Per-Ola Granberg and the Stockholm Endocrine Surgery group, together with the Nordic Surgical Association, described the role of surgeons' experience in the outcome of parathyroid surgery, several studies have highlighted this topic [10] and four studies have looked at a direct comparison between surgeon volume and parathyroidectomy outcomes.

Among these studies, there is the one by Stavrakis et al. [8], who evaluated the effect of surgeon volume on clinical and economic outcomes for thyroid, parathyroid and adrenal surgery using cross-sectional hospital data from both inpatient and outpatient surgeries in New York and Florida for a single year. They created six surgeon volume groups with a roughly equal distribution of cases, including those who performed 1–3, 4–8, 9–19, 20–50, 51–99, and ≥100 cases per year. It is to be noted that these numbers represent endocrine cases and not specifically parathyroid ones, but the parathyroid-specific data can be extrapolated. In total, 3412 parathyroid cases were performed in the study period, and they were more likely to be performed by high-volume surgeons. The overall complication rates were inversely related to volume, with complication rates—from lowest to highest surgeon volume groups—being 9.13%, 4.35%, 3.51%, 2.22%, 2.43% and 0.44%, respectively. Simply stated, the highest volume surgeons had the lowest complication rates. They also demonstrated a significant observed-to-expected complication ratio for both the lowest- and the highest-volume surgeons. Those who performed 1–3 endocrine cases per year had an observed-to-expected complication rate ratio of 1.82; on the other hand, those who performed 100 or more endocrine cases per year had an observed-to-expected complication rate ratio of 0.25 (both rate ratios referring to parathyroid cases).

Neychev et al. [40] evaluated the outcomes of four parathyroid surgeons practicing at a community hospital who were compared to an expert endocrine surgeon from a high-volume academic center; the study set out to assess whether a surgeon's operative volume is the most important factor affecting rates of cure and complications in parathyroid surgery. They evaluated patients undergoing an initial operation for primary hyperparathyroidism (PHPT) over a 12-year period at a community hospital, and over a 3-year period at an academic institution. The surgeons at the community hospital had an annual parathyroid procedure volume of 17 ± 8 cases, while at the academic institution the volume was 73 ± 26 cases. The findings showed that the rates of cure were 97% and 99%, respectively; in the community hospital group, 6 out of 204 (2.9%) patients required a second operation for persistent hyperparathyroidism, compared with 2 out of 218 (0.9%) patients in the academic hospital group. Importantly, although there was a notable difference in the operative volumes between the two groups, both were considered experienced parathyroid surgeons and had high cure rates with minimal complications. The authors thus concluded that some of the magnitude of case volume difference was due to a referral pattern toward the high-volume center, but also that experienced surgeons achieve excellent results in either setting, supporting the premise that surgeon volume outweighs hospital volume when analyzing parathyroid surgery outcomes.

Also the study by Meltzer et al. [41] had the same purpose. They compared a population of 2080 unique patients with a single parathyroid surgery performed over a 6-year period by surgeons who performed either 20 or less, or more than 40 parathyroid operations per year. They matched the cases to reach 547 matched pairs between the two groups. Interestingly, their study revealed excellent outcomes in parathyroid surgery without significant differences between the two groups. The overall complication rates were comparable, although slightly higher in the low-volume surgeon group (10.8% compared to 9.3%); rates of hypocalcemia were insignificantly higher in the high-volume surgeon group, at 1.6% compared to 1.3%. The only complication reaching statistical significance was vocal cord paralysis, which occurred at a rate of 1.6% in the low-volume group, compared to 0.2% in the high-volume group, but the high-volume surgeon group was also more likely to perform an outpatient procedure, 59.6% of cases, compared to 34.1%.

Also Sosa et al. [42] reported on outcomes in relation to surgeon volume, but their study was based on self-reported data from a survey of North American members of the American Association of Endocrine Surgeons. They demonstrated a significant variation in physician decision-making for the surgical management of PHPT based on surgeons' annual caseload. The surgical outcomes varied as well, both based on annual caseload, and when adjusted for years since training was completed. In general, though, regardless of years since completion of training, there was a significant difference in the complication rates after primary or remedial parathyroid surgery for those who perform less than 15 cases compared to those who perform 50 or more cases per year. While the reported complication rates were also higher for the intermediate group of 15–49 cases per year, neither adjusted nor unadjusted rates reached statistical significance. On the contrary, as for in-hospital postoperative mortality, the unadjusted rates were statistically significant for both the low- and intermediate-volume groups (at 1% and 0.73%, respectively), when compared to the high-volume group at 0.04%, although the adjusted rate differences were not significant.

The work by Dhillon et al. [43] is unique in their exploration of surgeon volume and outcomes. Indeed, although the only outcome described is vocal fold paresis, this study evaluated a single surgeon, and then stratified risk over the course of years of practice. For parathyroid cases alone, the rate of injury was very low, with only one injury in the total 374 cases performed over the study period, for an injury rate of 0.3%. Looking at the cases overall, they managed to show the impact of years of practice on a single surgeon's cumulative operative experience. While this stratification did not separate out parathyroid cases, it did show a change in the rate of injury as a function of years of practice: if the overall mean was 2.9%, the lowest nerve injury rate was observed during the final 2 years of the study, at 1.1%.

Further insights were provided in 2002, when Udelsman [44] published his series of 656 consecutive parathyroidectomies performed for PHPT over an 11-year period, inclusive of initial and reoperative cases. The complication rate was 2.3% (15 cases) including four recurrent laryngeal nerve injuries, of which two were in reoperative cases, two postoperative neck hematomas (of which one patient was on chronic anticoagulation), and two cases of postoperative hypocalcemia; moreover, in this series, three patients (0.5%) developed recurrent disease, of which two were reoperative cases. Additionally, this series demonstrated a clear financial benefit of minimally invasive parathyroidectomy when compared to conventional exploration. Operative time, anesthesia time, and hospital length of stay were all decreased in the minimally invasive compared with the conventional group, and each of these measures were associated with cost savings.

Expanding these data, in 2011 Udelsman et al. [45] reported 1650 consecutive parathyroidectomies performed by a single high-volume surgeon over a 19-year period. While the goal of the publication was to compare minimally invasive and conventional parathyroidectomy, it highlighted the parathyroid surgical outcomes for a single high-volume surgeon. It showed, indeed, an overall 98.5% cure rate including both conventional and focused interventions, with initial and remedial cases. The rate of complications was 2.1% overall, with the rate of recurrent laryngeal nerve injury, neck hematoma, and postoperative hypocalcemia each below 1%. Separating complications by initial surgical intervention and reoperative surgery, the complication rates were 1.8% and 3.8%, respectively, consistent with other studies showing higher complication rates in reoperative surgery. This series also demonstrated decreased costs in parathyroid surgery when resources exist for a focused approach. In the minimally invasive subgroup, indeed, the mean length of stay was 0.2 days with a median of 0 days, as 85% had outpatient surgery; in the conventional group, on the other hand, the mean length of stay was 1.3 days.

Reoperative parathyroid surgery has been evaluated independently in several series; some examples will follow.

Shen et al. [46] published a series of 102 patients who underwent reoperative parathyroidectomy for persistent or recurrent disease during a 10-year period. Remedial surgery proved curative in 95% of the cases, but one patient had permanent postoperative hypocalcemia after surgery, and one had permanent vocal cord paralysis.

Following the same line, Jaskowiak et al. [47] published a prospective study on 288 consecutive patients referred to the National Institutes of Health over a 13-year period, after at least one previous neck exploration for PHPT at another institution.

After excluding 66 patients due to a diagnosis of parathyroid cancer, multiple endocrine neoplasia type 1 or non-familial multigland hyperplasia, they analyzed the remaining 222 patients believed to have single gland disease; of these, 5% had three or more previous explorations, 17% had two previous exploration, and 78% had one previous exploration. The majority (92%) had one or more previous failed operations, whereas 8% were initially cured, but developed recurrent disease six or more months after surgery. Similar to the aforementioned study by Shen et al., the reoperative success rate was 94.1%, with 209 patients having a single successful exploration. Of the 13 operative failures, six underwent a second remedial operation during the study and were cured. The complications included six temporary and three permanent recurrent laryngeal nerve injuries, one permanent marginal mandibular nerve injury, three bleeds that required transfusion but not reoperation, and 61 cases of severe postoperative hypocalcemia. Of these 61 hypocalcemia cases, seven needed intravenous calcium, 42 required vitamin D supplementation, and 12 necessitated a delayed parathyroid autograft from cryopreserved tissue, though the autograft function was not reported.

Dealing specifically with reoperations, in 2006 Udelsman et al. [48] reported outcomes in 130 consecutive reoperative parathyroidectomies in 128 patients over a 15-year period. These patients included those with persistent PHPT after a failed exploration, recurrent PHPT, or newly developed PHPT in the setting of previous neck exploration—such as thyroidectomy—and was inclusive of patients with parathyroid carcinoma, multigland parathyroid hyperplasia, and familial hyperparathyroid syndromes. Even though the previous interventions varied, 13 had undergone two or more previous parathyroid explorations. In this series, the overall cure rate was 95%, thus in keeping with the previously mentioned studies; this rate is lower than that obtained with the initial procedures performed in the same period (i.e., 98%). There were seven cases in six patients who failed to achieve cure during remedial exploration (5%). Of these, four had multigland disease, one in the setting of multiple endocrine neoplasia 2A with previous total thyroidectomy, and one patient had a supernumerary gland (such cases had been excluded in the analysis by Jaskowiak et al. [47]). There were also four complications: three recurrent laryngeal nerve injuries and one mild stroke.

Interestingly, and providing a different kind of study sample, Tuggle et al. [49] evaluated pediatric surgical outcomes. High-volume surgeons were defined as those who performed over 30 annual cervical endocrine cases and averaged 72 per year. When compared with pediatric and other surgeons performing the same cases on the same patient subgroup, and without overlap, the high-volume surgeons had an overall complication rate of 8.7% compared to 13.4% and 13.2%, respectively, and an endocrine-specific complication rate of 5.6% compared to 11.0% and 9.5%, respectively.

Regarding parathyroid surgery, four studies [8, 37, 40, 42] offered a direct comparison between surgeon volume and outcomes, but they differed significantly in surgeon volume stratification. Indeed, though they demonstrated improved outcomes with increased surgeon volume, there was no clear volume threshold elucidated.

Self-reported survey data can be extrapolated to support the view that the ideal parathyroid surgeon is one who performs 50 or more cases per year [42]. However, most of the endpoints did not reach statistical significance for the intermediate group, and those who perform 15 or more cases per year have results comparable to those performing 50 or more. This suggests that surgeons who perform between one to two cases a month and those who perform one or more cases per week approach equivalency in outcomes.

In this regard, Stavrakis et al. [8] analyzed results of parathyroid surgery based on surgeon volume. The highest-volume surgeons, here defined as those performing over 100 endocrine cases per year, had a better outcome profile when compared to any of the lower-volume groups. On close analysis, however, this simplicity is blurred by the fact that the complication rates were similar for those performing 20–50 and 51–99 endocrine cases per year, and they were actually higher for those in the 51–99 case group. Thus, this report suggests that a surgeon volume of 100 or more annual cases is ideal, but one of 20 cases or more could be sufficient.

Similarly, Neychev et al. [40] examined surgeons performing around 17 versus 73 parathyroid cases a year and concluded that results were adequate in both groups, although there was a slightly higher failure rate in the lower volume group. Yet another time, this leans toward the determination that an annual parathyroid volume of 15–20 cases is sufficient.

Perhaps the most revealing information regarding outcomes in parathyroid surgery comes from the published individual series. These are greatly skewed towards high-volume parathyroid surgeons, and yet, even in these series, the volume of parathyroid surgery varies greatly, all with excellent results. Averaging volumes, rates vary from 23 to 87 parathyroid cases per year, with approximately 10 reoperative cases per year. As these publications cite data from some of the most experienced parathyroid surgeons, one could argue these are the ideal values; however, the volumes vary widely, and it may be unreasonable to impose these volume suggestions upon the majority of surgeons performing parathyroid surgery. In conclusion, the issue is that there is a paucity of data, and there are few publications demonstrating a consensus on the threshold case volume required to be an ideal parathyroid surgeon [10, 14].

10.4   Adrenal Surgery

The majority of adrenalectomies in the United States are performed by surgeons who do just one adrenalectomy per year [50, 51]. Several studies have sought to determine the association between operative volume and patient outcomes in adrenal surgery, but, given the overall rarity of adrenalectomies, most studies conducted in the United States are based on retrospective studies using state- and national-level databases. Most of these studies examine a few outcomes of interest, often including occurrence of ≥1 complications, length of stay, and cost of hospitalization. Initial studies of a volume-outcome relationship for adrenalectomy revealed conflicting results.

One of the first analyses to examine the volume-outcome association in adrenal surgery was the study conducted by Stavrakis et al. [8] on endocrine surgical procedures (thyroidectomy, parathyroidectomy, and adrenalectomy) based on data culled from New York and Florida state databases. The authors grouped surgeons into 1 of 6 groups based on their cumulative volume of endocrine-specific procedures performed during 2002: group A, 1–3 operations annually; B, 4–8; C, 9–19; D, 20–50; E, 51–99; F, ≥100. When the outcomes of patients who underwent adrenalectomy were examined, the study found no association between surgeon volume and complication rates (observed-to-expected ratios: 1.04, 0.84, 1.00, 1.67, 0.00, 0.83 for groups A to F, respectively, $p > 0.05$). Interestingly, though, each unit increase in surgeon volume was associated with a 0.28-day decrease in hospital length of stay ($p < 0.001$), and with a decrease in cost equal to $1472 ($p < 0.01$). However, the study had some key limitations: first of all, surgeon volume was cumulative for all endocrine procedures, and thus not restricted to adrenalectomy; data were derived from just two US states, limiting generalizability; and the study did not examine surgical approach (open vs. laparoscopic). Furthermore, the study did not adjust for hospital characteristics, such as teaching status and location (rural versus urban), which might influence patient outcomes.

Some of these limitations were overcome by another study by Gallagher et al. [52], also published in 2007: in this paper, they retrospectively analyzed hospital discharges from a database maintained by the Florida Agency for Health Care Administration, for 1816 patients who underwent adrenalectomy in the 1998–2005 period. Surgeons were assigned to one of four quartile groups based on their annual volume of adrenalectomies (1, 2, 3–6, ≥7 adrenalectomies/year). Again, no association was found between surgeon volume and postoperative complication rates (20%, 14%, 20%, 46%, for the successive surgeon volume groups, $p = 0.871$), but there was a lower mean hospital stay with increasing surgeon volume (7, 6, 7, and 5 days, respectively, $p < 0.001$).

However, both these inaugural studies likely lacked generalizability, since data were derived from only one or two states.

This situation was to be changed in 2009, thanks to a study by Park et al. [50], who examined a total of 3144 adrenalectomies, this time captured in the Nationwide Inpatient Sample (NIS; 1999–2005). First, the authors stratified surgeon volume based on quartiles: the top quartile (based on the performance of ≥4 adrenalectomies per year) was defined as high-volume, and the lower quartiles (<4 adrenalectomies per year) were defined as low-volume. The authors found that high-volume surgeons performed more bilateral adrenalectomies and used a laparoscopic approach more often; these surgeons operated more frequently at urban and teaching hospitals. Differently from previous studies, this one showed that adrenalectomies performed by low-volume surgeons were associated with a higher complication rate (18.3 vs. 11.3%, $p < 0.001$) and longer length of stay (5.5 vs. 3.9 days, $p < 0.001$) compared to those performed by high-volume surgeons. Differences in mean cost of hospitalization were not significant ($11,000 vs. $12,600 for high- vs. low-volume surgeons, respectively, but with $p = 0.06$). Importantly, this was the first study dealing with the adrenalectomy volume-outcome relationship using national-level data;

it was also the first to provide population-level evidence for a lower risk of complications when adrenalectomy is performed by high-volume surgeons. The study also confirmed the results of previous studies [52] which had shown a shorter duration of hospital stay for patients undergoing adrenalectomy by high volume surgeons. However, the study was limited in its ability to delineate the surgical approach.

Later, also Hauch et al. [53] provided up-to-date results using data from the Nationwide Inpatient Sample (2003–2009), for a total of 7829 adrenalectomies included in their study. Surgeon volume was analyzed based on a quartile distribution: low (1 adrenalectomy/year), intermediate (2–5 adrenalectomies/year), and high (>5 adrenalectomies/year). In bearing with the preceding study, the authors found that complication rates for low- and intermediate-volume surgeons were 18.8% and 14.6%, respectively, and that both groups had significantly higher complication rates than high-volume surgeons (11.6%, $p < 0.001$). Once again, the length of stay was also shorter when adrenalectomy was performed by a high-volume surgeon (high 2.7 ± 0.2 days vs. low 4.2 ± 0.1 days, $p < 0.001$). Similar to Park et al. [50], the authors found that surgeon volume was inversely associated with complication risks in multivariate regression modeling. In contrast to Park et al.'s results [50], this study reported significantly lower charges for high-volume surgeons compared to lower-volume groups ($p < 0.05$) when patients did not experience any complications ($27,324.00 ± 1882.05 vs. $33,499.00 ± 1062.81, $p = 0.001$), but the association was not significant, with occurrence of ≥1 complications ($70,523 vs. $78,299, $p < 0.05$). Of note, the use of hospital charges in the Nationwide Inpatient Sample is problematic, since charges are unadjusted for pertinent cost-to-charge ratios and inflation rates.

Yet another study, by Al-Qurayshi et al. [54], utilized data from the Nationwide Inpatient Sample (2003–2009) to examine 7045 patients who underwent adrenalectomy, this time with the specific aim of determining cost differences related to surgical volume; the authors also estimated potential cost savings based on surgeon volume, extrapolating their findings to a national level. Surgeon volume was classified based on the annual number of adrenalectomies performed by each surgeon: low-volume (≤25th percentile, 1 adrenalectomy/year), intermediate-volume (>25th to ≤75th percentiles, 2–6 adrenalectomies/year), and high-volume surgeons (>75th percentile, ≥7 adrenalectomies/year). The study showed that adrenalectomies performed by low-volume surgeons were associated with a higher risk of postoperative complications (adjusted OR 1.66, 95% CI 1.23–2.24). Then, after having built a hypothetical statistical model, the authors calculated incremental cost savings of 7.7% and 8.1% if all adrenalectomies performed by low-volume surgeons were selectively referred to intermediate- and high-volume surgeons, respectively. The highest cost savings (32.4%) were calculated for patients with a Charlson comorbidity score >2 who underwent adrenalectomy by a high-volume surgeon. Additionally, based on a conservative assumption that 5000 adrenalectomies are performed in the United States every year, the authors extrapolated hypothetical cost savings of $19.8 million if intermediate-volume surgeons performed cases done by low-volume surgeons, and cost savings of $24.8 million if these patients were treated by high-volume surgeons. This study thus demonstrated that improved clinical outcomes of high-volume adrenal surgeons might also have a potentially large economic implication.

Furthermore, a study by Lindeman et al. [55] showed a significant association between surgeon volume and mortality following adrenalectomy. The study analyzed adrenalectomies captured in the New York Statewide Planning and Research Cooperative System from 2000 to 2014. High surgeon volume was defined using a threshold of ≥4 adrenalectomies per year, and the volume threshold was chosen based on Park et al.'s [50] data. The authors found that patients of high-volume surgeons experienced significantly lower mortality (0.56% vs. 1.25%, $p = 0.004$) and a lower overall rate of complications (10.2% vs. 16.4%, $p < 0.001$) compared to those of low-volume surgeons. It is important to note that, after risk adjustment, low-surgeon volume proved to be an independent predictor of patients experiencing an inpatient complication (OR 0.96, $p = 0.002$).

Further confirming these findings, Palazzo et al. [56] examined 795 adult adrenalectomies performed by 222 different surgeons in the United Kingdom (2013–2014). Only 36 (16%) adrenal surgeons performed ≥6 adrenalectomies, which was the definition of a high-volume surgeon used in the study; also, a total of 186 surgeons (84%) performed a median of one adrenalectomy per year. The study showed that length of stay and readmission rates within 30 days of surgery were compromised when adrenalectomy was performed by low-volume surgeons (60% longer and 47% higher, respectively). Thus, the authors concluded that, in the United Kingdom, higher volume surgeons best perform adrenal surgery in centers with a dedicated adrenal multidisciplinary team expert in all aspects of care.

These findings are consistent with those of a Spanish study [57] in which high-volume surgeons (≥5 adrenalectomies per year) were found to have higher rates of performing a laparoscopic approach (91.9% vs. 74.5%, $p = 0.03$), lower rates of in-hospital complications (4.0% vs. 14.8%, $p = 0.02$), and also shorter length of stay (3.9 vs. 5.3 days, $p < 0.001$).

Although the reported studies show a general coherence, the problem is that volume thresholds for adrenalectomy are often arbitrarily selected; this makes comparison across studies difficult. To address this lack of uniformity, Anderson et al. [58] used sophisticated analyses with restricted cubic splines to determine the appropriate adrenalectomy volume threshold that can be used to define a surgeon as high-volume. The authors examined the National Inpatient Sample (1998–2009), abstracting 6712 patients who underwent adrenalectomies at 687 hospitals by 3496 surgeons; median annual surgeon volume was one case. Although the study did not adjust for surgical approach, it showed that the likelihood of experiencing a complication decreased with increasing annual surgeon volume up to 5.6 cases; thus, lower volume surgeons were deemed to be those who performed <6 adrenalectomies per year. When outcomes were re-analyzed based on this binary volume stratification, and after multivariate adjustment, the authors found that patients undergoing adrenalectomy by low-volume surgeons (<6 cases/year) were more likely to experience complications (OR 1.71, 95% CI 1.27–2.31, $p = 0.005$), have a longer hospital stay (RR 1.46, 95% CI 1.25–1.70, $p = 0.003$), and at increased cost (+26.2%, 95% CI 12.6–39.9, $p = 0.02$). Thus, the study established that high-volume adrenal surgeons

achieve improved outcomes compared with surgeons who perform <6 adrenalectomies per year. It also confirmed the results of an earlier study by Lindeman et al.
[55], which had shown an association between surgeon volume and postoperative
mortality after adrenalectomy (0.6% vs. 2.4% for low vs. high volume surgeons,
respectively, $p < 0.001$).

To also address the question of the different techniques, Faiena et al. [59] studied
8831 patients who underwent open, laparoscopic, or robotic adrenalectomy for
benign or malignant disease in the Premier Hospital Database (2003–2013). In the
end, the authors found no significant difference in complication rates or operative
times based on surgical specialty.

But there is more: indeed, it should be noted that, compared to studies focused
on surgeon volume, those that have studied a hospital adrenalectomy volume-
outcome association are comparatively fewer in number, more heterogeneous in
patients' and providers' characteristics, and more often specific to surgical technique or disease process. The studies that have evaluated the association between
hospital adrenalectomy volume and postoperative outcomes have yielded divergent
results. To complicate matters further, in contrast to high-volume surgeons performing adrenalectomies, a high-volume adrenalectomy center is not currently
defined yet.

One of the studies dealing with this topic was the one by Bergamini et al. [60];
they analyzed 833 adrenalectomies captured in the Italian Registry of Endoscopic
Surgery-Adrenalectomy database (2000–2009). Then, surgical centers were arbitrarily divided into "referral centers" with >30 adrenalectomies and "non-referral
centers" with <30 adrenalectomies performed. Results showed that patients
undergoing surgery at referral centers had lower rates of conversions to laparotomy (1.6% vs. 6.0%, $p = 0.003$) and postoperative complications (4.8% vs. 22.0%,
$p < 0.001$).

These results are similar to those of a study of more than 8000 patients who
underwent adrenalectomy in New York, New Jersey, and Pennsylvania [61]. Volume
was stratified based on quintiles that were created using 1996 hospital volumes:
very-low-volume hospital (VLVH), 0–1 cases; low-volume hospital (LVH), 2–3
cases; moderate-volume hospital (MVH), 4–6 cases; high-volume hospital (HVH),
7–14 cases; and very-high-volume hospital (VHVH), ≥15 cases per year. The
authors found that patients were less likely to die when treated at VHVHs than at
VLVHs (OR 0.38, 95% CI 0.19–0.75, $p = 0.006$). Moreover, a shorter hospital
length of stay was associated with each increasing volume quintile. When controlling for year treated, a median difference of 1.75 days (95% CI 1.80–1.69, $p < 0.001$)
of hospital stay was noted in the VHVH cohort compared to the VLVH group.

In contrast to these results, though, Murphy et al.'s [62] analysis of more than
40,000 adrenalectomies captured in the Nationwide Inpatient Sample (1998–2006)
found no significant difference in risk of complications based on hospital volume;
this finding was noted in both univariate and multivariate analyses.

The relative influence of surgeon vs. hospital volume on patient outcomes
remains unresolved, as few studies have included both surgeon and hospital volume
together in their analyses.

For instance, a study by Al-Qurayshi et al. [54] showed that, when controlling for multiple factors, including surgeon volume, patients managed in low- (1–3 adrenal-ectomies/year) or intermediate-volume hospitals (4–64 adrenalectomies/year) did not have a statistically significant difference in risk of postoperative complications compared to those managed in high-volume hospitals (>75th percentile or ≥65 adrenalectomies/year) ([low-volume hospital: OR 1.09, 95% CI 0.73–1.63, $p = 0.67$] [intermediate-volume hospital: OR 1.04, 95% CI 0.78–1.40, $p = 0.79$]).

This finding echoes Hauch et al.'s [53] analysis of the Nationwide Inpatient Sample, in which hospital adrenalectomy volume impacted on the risk of postopera-tive complications in univariate analyses ($p = 0.004$) but then lost significance in multivariate analyses after controlling for several factors, including surgeon volume.

However, volume-outcome studies that take into consideration surgical tech-nique tend to assess hospital rather than surgeon volume for that specific technique; a problem is that thresholds for volume are commonly arbitrary.

One example is the study by Greco et al. [63] about 363 patients who underwent laparoscopic adrenalectomy at 23 centers in Germany. In this analysis, centers were stratified into three groups according to their laparoscopic adrenalectomy experi-ence: group A (<10/year), group B (10–20/year) and group C (>20/year). Although complications were not analyzed in the study, when groups A, B, and C were com-pared, mean operative time proved to be significantly shorter at higher-volume cen-ters (105.4 vs. 116.5 vs. 159.9 min $p = 0.013$) but there was no difference in hospital length of stay (6.9 vs. 7.1 vs. 7.4 days, $p = 0.942$).

Further insights were provided by a similar study by Villar et al. [57]: they ana-lyzed 155 adrenalectomies performed in 2008 in surgical departments in Spain, high-volume centers were defined as those with an annual volume ≥10 adrenalecto-mies, while low volume centers were those with an annual volume <10 adrenalec-tomies that year. The authors found that high-volume centers were more likely to use laparoscopy (92.2% vs. 75.6% $p = 0.008$), treat malignant lesions (20.7% vs. 8.9%, $p = 0.03$), and have a shorter length of hospital stay (3.7 vs. 5.5 days, $p < 0.001$). Yet, although high-volume centers had lower rates of conversion to lapa-rotomy, fewer postoperative complications and reoperations, these differences were nonsignificant, likely due to low statistical power. In addition, adjusted analyses to adequately delineate the independent impact of surgeon vs. hospital volume were not performed.

A remarkable study is the one by Gratian et al. [64]: it is, indeed, one of the few focusing on a specific disease process—adrenocortical carcinoma (ACC). In their study, 2765 patients with ACC were identified from 1046 facilities participating in the National Cancer Database (1998–2011). High-volume centers were defined by a volume of ≥4 cases of ACC annually, which corresponded to the 90th percentile of case volume in the study cohort. All other facilities were considered low-volume centers. From a surgical perspective, patients treated at high-volume centers experi-enced higher rates of adrenalectomy (78.8% vs. 73.4%), radical resection (17.3% vs. 13.9%), regional lymph node evaluation (23.2% vs. 18.8%), and chemotherapy, including mitotane (43.8% vs. 31.0%, all $p < 0.05$), compared to patients treated at low-volume centers. There were no significant differences in median length of stay

(5 days), 30-day readmissions (4.0% for high-volume centers vs. 3.9% for low-volume centers), or 30-day postoperative mortality (1.9% for high-volume centers vs. 3.7% for low-volume centers). Results showed that, despite more aggressive operations, fewer positive surgical margins, and more adjuvant treatment at high-volume centers, overall survival did not differ based on hospital volume.

Following this line, Kerkhofs et al. [65] evaluated patients with stages I–III ACC followed in the National Cancer Registry in the Netherlands. However, their results differed from those of the aforementioned study by Gratian et al. [64]: indeed, 5-year overall survival was improved for patients undergoing surgery in a Dutch Adrenal Network (DAN) hospital compared to those having surgery in a non-DAN hospital (63% vs. 42%, $p = 0.044$ in unadjusted analyses; hazard ratio: 1.96, $p = 0.047$ in adjusted analyses).

Similarly, in an Italian multicentric series [66], performance of aggressive surgery was more likely at high-volume centers (lymphadenectomy rate: 22% vs. 7.7% at low-volume centers, $p < 0.01$; multi-organ resection rate: 24% vs. 8% at low-volume centers, $p < 0.01$). On the other hand, the proportion of patients who underwent laparoscopic resection for ACC was higher at low-volume compared to high-volume centers (19.7% vs. 8.7%, respectively, $p < 0.05$). Furthermore, local and distant ACC recurrences occurred more frequently in patients who underwent their initial operation at low-volume centers, and the mean time to recurrence was shorter at low-volume centers (10.1 ± 7.5 months vs. 25.2 ± 28.1 months $p < 0.001$). Median disease-specific survival was 63 months at high-volume centers, and 32 months at low-volume centers, with median overall survival being 24 and 15 months, respectively; however, these differences were not statistically significant, likely due to small sample size.

Following this line, a recent meta-analysis [67] examined contemporary management of ACC by including five studies that presented data on provider volume. Overall, the authors found that high-volume centers performed more aggressive, open surgery for ACC, and their patients experienced lower rates of local and distant recurrence, as well as a longer time to recurrence. However, the findings of the meta-analysis were once again limited by the fact that a threshold for high hospital volume was not defined; the meta-analysis also had significant data heterogeneity, as well as an overall low level of evidence.

10.5 Surgery for Gastroenteropancreatic Neuroendocrine Neoplasms

Because of the low incidence and the clinical and biological heterogeneity of gastroenteropancreatic neuroendocrine neoplasms, to date no studies have evaluated their outcomes in terms of surgeon volume and center volume. However, a recent survey by a working group of the European Society of Endocrine Surgeons [14] concluded that, due to the low incidence and broad range (of manifestations/clinical presentations) of gastroenteropancreatic neuroendocrine tumors (GEP-NET), a minimal annual caseload of 5 GEP-NET operations is required in order to obtain appropriate specialized knowledge in their peri- and intraoperative management.

10.6 Conclusion

In conclusion, there is considerable evidence supporting an operative volume-outcome association in endocrine surgery; moreover, evidence in favor of improved patient outcomes is stronger for high surgeon volume as compared to high hospital volume. High surgeon volume may be a proxy for advanced surgical skill and perhaps for diligence in following established clinical guidelines, such that improved patient outcomes are not only a reflection of technical ability, but also of an evidence-based multidisciplinary approach to patient care.

References

1. Luft HS. The relation between surgical volume and mortality: an exploration of causal factors and alternative models. Med Care. 1980;18(9):940–59.
2. Luft HS, Bunker JP, Enthoven AC. Should operations be regionalized? The empirical relation between surgical volume and mortality. N Engl J Med. 1979;301(25):1364–9.
3. Hannan EL, Radzyner M, Rubin D, et al. The influence of hospital and surgeon volume on in-hospital mortality for colectomy, gastrectomy, and lung lobectomy in patients with cancer. Surgery. 2002;131(1):6–15.
4. Dudley RA, Johansen KL, Brand R, et al. Selective referral to high-volume hospitals: estimating potentially avoidable deaths. JAMA. 2000;283(9):1159–66.
5. Bach PB, Cramer LD, Schrag D, et al. The influence of hospital volume on survival after resection for lung cancer. N Engl J Med. 2001;345(3):181–8.
6. Birkmeyer JD, Stukel TA, Siewers AE, et al. Surgeon volume and operative mortality in the United States. N Engl J Med. 2003;349:2117–27.
7. Halm EA, Lee C, Chassin MR. How is volume related to quality in health care? A systematic review of the research literature. Ann Intern Med. 2002;137:511–20.
8. Stavrakis AI, Ituarte PH, Ko CY, Yeh MW. Surgeon volume as a predictor of outcomes in inpatient and outpatient endocrine surgery. Surgery. 2007;142(6):887–99.
9. Chowdhury MM, Dagash H, Pierro A. A systematic review of the impact of volume of surgery and specialization on patient outcome. Br J Surg. 2007;94(2):145–61.
10. Erinjeri NJ, Udelsman R. Volume-outcome relationship in parathyroid surgery. Best Pract Res Clin Endocrinol Metab. 2019;33(5):101287. https://doi.org/10.1016/j.beem.2019.06.003.
11. Aspinall S, Oweis D, Chadwick D. Effect of surgeons' annual operative volume on the risk of permanent hypoparathyroidism, recurrent laryngeal nerve palsy and haematoma following thyroidectomy: analysis of United Kingdom registry of endocrine and thyroid surgery (UKRETS). Langenbeck's Arch Surg. 2019;404(4):421–30.
12. Jakob DA, Riss P, Scheuba C, et al. Association of surgical volume and quality management in thyroid surgery: a two-nation multicenter study. World J Surg. 2019;43(9):2218–27.
13. Kazaure HS, Sosa JA. Volume–outcome relationship in adrenal surgery: a review of existing literature. Best Pract Res Clin Endocrinol Metab. 2019;33(5):101296. https://doi.org/10.1016/j.beem.2019.101296.
14. Musholt TJ, Bränström R, Kaderli RM, et al. Accreditation of endocrine surgery units. Langenbeck's Arch Surg. 2019;404(7):779–93. https://doi.org/10.1007/s00423-019-01820-y.

15. Sosa JA, Bowman HM, Tielsch JM, et al. The importance of surgeon experience for clinical and economic outcomes from thyroidectomy. Ann Surg. 1998;228(3):320–30.
16. Dralle H, Sekulla C, Haerting J, et al. Risk factors of paralysis and functional outcome after recurrent laryngeal nerve monitoring in thyroid surgery. Surgery. 2004;136(6):1310–22.
17. Gourin CG, Tufano RP, Forastiere AA, et al. Volume-based trends in thyroid surgery. Arch Otolaryngol Head Neck Surg. 2010;136(12):1191–8.
18. Kandil E, Noureldine SI, Abbas A, Tufano RP. The impact of surgical volume on patient outcomes following thyroid surgery. Surgery. 2013;154(6):1346–52; discussion 1352–3.
19. Loyo M, Tufano RP, Gourin CG. National trends in thyroid surgery and the effect of volume on short-term outcomes. Laryngoscope. 2013;123(8):2056–63.
20. Adkisson CD, Howell GM, McCoy KL, et al. Surgeon volume and adequacy of thyroidectomy for differentiated thyroid cancer. Surgery. 2014;156(6):1453–9; discussion 1460.
21. Hauch A, Al-Qurayshi Z, Randolph G, Kandil E. Total thyroidectomy is associated with increased risk of complications for low- and high-volume surgeons. Ann Surg Oncol. 2014;21(12):3844–52.
22. Nouraei SA, Virk JS, Middleton SE, et al. A national analysis of trends, outcomes and volume–outcome relationships in thyroid surgery. Clin Otolaryngol. 2017;42(2):354–65.
23. Adam MA, Thomas S, Youngwirth L, et al. Is there a minimum number of thyroidectomies a surgeon should perform to optimize patient outcomes? Ann Surg. 2017;265(2):402–7.
24. Gharib H, Papini E, Garber JR, et al. American Association of Clinical Endocrinologists, American college of endocrinology, and Associazione Medici Endocrinologi medical guidelines for clinical practice for the diagnosis and management of thyroid nodules—2016 update. Endocr Pract. 2016;22(5):622–39.
25. Haugen BR, Alexander EK, Bible KC, et al. 2015 American Thyroid Association Management guidelines for adult patients with thyroid nodules and differentiated thyroid cancer: the American Thyroid Association Guidelines Task Force on thyroid nodules and differentiated thyroid cancer. Thyroid. 2016;26(1):1–133.
26. Pacini F, Castagna MG, Brilli L, Pentheroudakis G, ESMO Guidelines Working Group. Thyroid cancer: ESMO Clinical practice guidelines for diagnosis, treatment and follow-up. Ann Oncol. 2012;23(Suppl 7):vii110–9.
27. Dralle H, Musholt TJ, Schabram J, et al. German Association of Endocrine Surgeons practice guideline for the surgical management of malignant thyroid tumors. Langenbeck's Arch Surg. 2013;398(3):347–75.
28. Harris PE. The management of thyroid cancer in adults: a review of new guidelines. Clin Med (Lond). 2002;2(2):144–6.
29. Pitoia F, Ward L, Wohllk N, et al. Recommendations of the Latin American Thyroid Society on diagnosis and management of differentiated thyroid cancer. Arq Bras Endocrinol Metabol. 2009;53(7):884–7.
30. Martínez Trufero J, Capdevila J, Cruz JJ, Isla D. SEOM clinical guidelines for the treatment of thyroid cancer. Clin Transl Oncol. 2011;13(8):574–9.
31. Links TP, Huysmans DA, Smit JW, et al. Guideline "Differentiated thyroid carcinoma", including diagnosis of thyroid nodules. Ned Tijdschr Geneeskd. 2007;151(32):1777–82. [Article in Dutch].
32. Thomusch O, Machens A, Sekulla C, et al. Multivariate analysis of risk factors for postoperative complications in benign goiter surgery: prospective multicenter study in Germany. World J Surg. 2000;24(11):1335–41.
33. Mitchell J, Milas M, Barbosa G, et al. Avoidable reoperations for thyroid and parathyroid surgery: effect of hospital volume. Surgery. 2008;144(6):899–907.
34. Duclos A, Peix J-L, Colin C, et al. Influence of experience on performance of individual surgeons in thyroid surgery: prospective cross sectional multicentre study. BMJ. 2012;344:d8041. https://doi.org/10.1136/bmj.d8041.
35. González-Sánchez C, Franch-Arcas G, Gómez-Alonso A. Morbidity following thyroid surgery: does surgeon volume matter? Langenbeck's Arch Surg. 2013;398(3):419–22.

36. Al-Qurayshi Z, Robins R, Hauch A, et al. Association of surgeon volume with outcomes and cost savings following thyroidectomy: a national forecast. JAMA Otolaryngol Head Neck Surg. 2016;142(1):32–9.
37. Meltzer C, Klau M, Gurushanthaiah D, et al. Surgeon volume in thyroid surgery: surgical efficiency, outcomes, and utilization. Laryngoscope. 2016;126(11):2630–9.
38. Liang TJ, Liu SI, Mok KT, Shi HY. Associations of volume and thyroidectomy outcomes: a nationwide study with systematic review and meta-analysis. Otolaryngol Head Neck Surg. 2016;155(1):65–75.
39. Youngwirth LM, Adam MA, Scheri RP, et al. Patients treated at low-volume centers have higher rates of incomplete resection and compromised outcomes: analysis of 31,129 patients with papillary thyroid cancer. Ann Surg Oncol. 2016;23(2):403–9.
40. Neychev VK, Ghanem M, Blackwood SL, et al. Parathyroid surgery can be safely performed in a community hospital by experienced parathyroid surgeons: a retrospective cohort study. Int J Surg. 2016;27:72–6.
41. Meltzer C, Klau M, Gurushanthaiah D, et al. Surgeon volume in parathyroid surgery—surgical efficiency, outcomes, and utilization. JAMA Otolaryngol Neck Surg. 2017;143(8):843.
42. Sosa JA, Powe NR, Levine MA, et al. Profile of a clinical practice: thresholds for surgery and surgical outcomes for patients with primary hyperparathyroidism: a national survey of endocrine surgeons. J Clin Endocrinol Metab. 1998;83(8):2658–65.
43. Dhillon VK, Rettig E, Noureldine SI, et al. The incidence of vocal fold motion impairment after primary thyroid and parathyroid surgery for a single high-volume academic surgeon determined by pre- and immediate post-operative fiberoptic laryngoscopy. Int J Surg. 2018;56:73–8.
44. Udelsman R. Six hundred fifty-six consecutive explorations for primary hyperparathyroidism. Ann Surg. 2002;235(5):665–70; discussion 670–2.
45. Udelsman R, Lin Z, Donovan P. The superiority of minimally invasive parathyroidectomy based on 1650 consecutive patients with primary hyperparathyroidism. Ann Surg. 2011;253(3):585–91.
46. Shen W, Düren M, Morita E, et al. Reoperation for persistent or recurrent primary hyperparathyroidism. Arch Surg. 1996;131(8):861–9.
47. Jaskowiak N, Norton JA, Alexander HR, et al. A prospective trial evaluating a standard approach to reoperation for missed parathyroid adenoma. Ann Surg. 1996;224(3):308–20; discussion 320–1.
48. Udelsman R, Donovan PI. Remedial parathyroid surgery: changing trends in 130 consecutive cases. Ann Surg. 2006;244(3):471–9.
49. Tuggle CT, Roman SA, Wang TS, et al. Pediatric endocrine surgery: who is operating on our children? Surgery. 2008;144(6):869–77.
50. Park HS, Roman SA, Sosa JA. Outcomes from 3144 adrenalectomies in the United States: which matters more, surgeon volume or specialty? Arch Surg. 2009;144(11):1060–7.
51. Saunders BD, Wainess RM, Dimick JB, et al. Who performs endocrine operations in the United States? Surgery. 2003;134(6):924–31; discussion 931.
52. Gallagher SF, Wahi M, Haines KL, et al. Trends in adrenalectomy rates, indications, and physician volume: a statewide analysis of 1816 adrenalectomies. Surgery. 2007;142(6):1011–21.
53. Hauch A, Al-Qurayshi Z, Kandil E. Factors associated with higher risk of complications after adrenal surgery. Ann Surg Oncol. 2015;22(1):103–10.
54. Al-Qurayshi Z, Robins R, Buell J, Kandil E. Surgeon volume impact on outcomes and cost of adrenal surgeries. Eur J Surg Oncol. 2016;42(10):1483–90.
55. Lindeman B, Hashimoto DA, Bababekov YJ, et al. Fifteen years of adrenalectomies: impact of specialty training and operative volume. Surgery. 2018;163(1):150–6.
56. Palazzo F, Dickinson A, Phillips B, et al. Adrenal surgery in England: better outcomes in high-volume practices. Clin Endocrinol. 2016;85(1):17–20.
57. Villar JM, Moreno P, Ortega J, et al. Results of adrenal surgery. Data of a Spanish National Survey. Langenbeck's Arch Surg. 2010;395(7):837–43.

58. Anderson KL, Thomas SM, Adam MA, et al. Each procedure matters: threshold for surgeon volume to minimize complications and decrease cost associated with adrenalectomy. Surgery. 2018;163(1):157–64.
59. Faiena I, Tabakin A, Leow J, et al. Adrenalectomy for benign and malignant disease: utilization and outcomes by surgeon specialty and surgical approach from 2003–2013. Can J Urol. 2017;24(5):8990–7.
60. Bergamini C, Martellucci J, Tozzi F, Valeri A. Complications in laparoscopic adrenalectomy: the value of experience. Surg Endosc. 2011;25(12):3845–51.
61. Simhan J, Smaldone MC, Canter DJ, et al. Trends in regionalization of adrenalectomy to higher volume surgical centers. J Urol. 2012;188(2):377–82.
62. Murphy MM, Witkowski ER, Ng SC, et al. Trends in adrenalectomy: a recent national review. Surg Endosc. 2010;24(10):2518–26.
63. Greco F, Hoda MR, Rassweiler J, et al. Laparoscopic adrenalectomy in urological centres— the experience of the German Laparoscopic Working Group. BJU Int. 2011;108(10):1646–51.
64. Gratian L, Pura J, Dinan M, et al. Treatment patterns and outcomes for patients with adrenocortical carcinoma associated with hospital case volume in the United States. Ann Surg Oncol. 2014;21(11):3509–14.
65. Kerkhofs TM, Verhoeven RH, Bonjer HJ, et al. Surgery for adrenocortical carcinoma in the Netherlands: analysis of the national cancer registry data. Eur J Endocrinol. 2013;169(1):83–9.
66. Lombardi CP, Raffaelli M, Boniardi M, et al. Adrenocortical carcinoma: effect of hospital volume on patient outcome. Langenbeck's Arch Surg. 2012;397(2):201–7.
67. Langenhuijsen J, Birtle A, Klatte T, et al. Surgical management of adrenocortical carcinoma: impact of laparoscopic approach, lymphadenectomy, and surgical volume on outcomes—a systematic review and meta-analysis of the current literature. Eur Urol Focus. 2016;1(3):241–50.

The Specific Role of Minimally Invasive Robotic Digestive Surgery

11

Felice Borghi, Paolo Pietro Bianchi, Luigi Pugliese, Andrea Peri, Giampaolo Formisano, and Andrea Pietrabissa

11.1 Introduction

The widespread diffusion of robotic surgical platforms over the last decades has led to its progressive implementation into several fields of surgery. Today, almost every known surgical procedure has been attempted with robotic assistance proving the feasibility and safety of the technology when performed by experienced surgeons. Despite the technological advantages of the available platforms which make the mastery of the robotic approach easier and faster to achieve than conventional minimally invasive techniques, the issues of training, credentialing and development of defined structured programs for robotic surgery are still under lively debate. Recent reports from different countries have shown a clear trend towards the decentralization of robotic procedures to an increasing number of centers each performing small numbers of cases per year; these low-volume centers, responsible for the majority of robotic procedures that are performed yearly in many countries, are associated with increased morbidity and mortality of patients operated on with the robotic

F. Borghi
General and Oncologic Surgical Unit, Department of Surgery,
Santa Croce e Carle Hospital, Cuneo, Italy
e-mail: borghi.f@ospedale.cuneo.it

P. P. Bianchi · G. Formisano
Division of General and Minimally Invasive Surgery, Department of Surgery
South-East Tuscany, Misericordia Hospital, Grosseto, Italy
e-mail: bianchippt@gmail.com; giampaolo.formisano@uslsudest.toscana.it

L. Pugliese · A. Peri
Department of Surgery, Fondazione IRCCS Policlinico San Matteo, Pavia, Italy
e-mail: luipugliese@gmail.com

A. Pietrabissa (✉)
Department of Surgery, Fondazione IRCCS Policlinico San Matteo,
University of Pavia, Pavia, Italy
e-mail: a.pietrabissa@smatteo.pv.it

© Springer Nature Switzerland AG 2021
M. Montorsi (ed.), *Volume-Outcome Relationship in Oncological Surgery*,
Updates in Surgery, https://doi.org/10.1007/978-3-030-51806-6_11

approach as compared with open or laparoscopic surgery. In addition, greater conversion rates, worse oncological outcomes, longer hospital stays and higher costs have been recorded for low-volume centers compared with high-volume ones. This reflects, on the one hand, the lack of the surgical team's experience and, on the other, poor availability of defined pathways and resources to deal with higher complication rates. The available data on the learning curve of robotic operations are extremely heterogeneous even when considering a specific procedure, though most of the authors agree that the plateau for surgical proficiency is reached much earlier than with laparoscopy. Moreover, the latter approach is not necessarily a mandatory requirement to succeed in performing safe and effective robotic interventions, which can be done with satisfactory outcomes even without prior laparoscopic experience; skilled laparoscopic surgeons may have a shorter learning curve at the robotic console, if any, and cope with more complex cases from the start. However, structured training programs and proctorship by expert robotic surgeons are the key steps to quickly master the technique at any level and to limit the related risks.

The largest published series for specific robotic applications mostly come from single surgeons or single institutions with vast experience in the field, making the results hard to compare and analyze with those of other series. Nevertheless, the enabling nature of robotic surgical platforms towards complex minimally invasive procedures (namely esophageal, pancreatic, or rectal resections) and the increasing evidence of improved outcomes of the robotic approach compared to standard laparoscopy for some of those procedures (lower conversion rate and shorter hospital stay) support the need to optimize the use of this costly technology within the healthcare system. Despite the evident lack of up-to-date information on the actual distribution of robotic procedures in Italy, centralization of patients who may benefit from the robotic approach to high-volume institutions according to the hub-spoke model should be encouraged by healthcare providers in order to maximize the cost-effectiveness of robotic surgery.

11.2   Robotic Esophageal and Gastric Oncologic Surgery

Since the first robotic esophagectomy and gastrectomy for cancer were performed in the early 2000s, no publications exist concerning the definition of hospital and surgeon volumes related to surgical and oncologic outcomes, as instead clearly demonstrated for open surgery. Moreover, in Italy data about robotic surgery are not among the indicators of the Italian National Agency for Regional Health Services (AGENAS). Despite the lack of this information, robotic upper gastrointestinal oncologic surgery is increasing in terms of volume of cases (Figs. 11.1 and 11.2) and number of published series.

In this situation we need to define, as a minimum requirement, a correct learning curve pathway to be able to guarantee at least the same standards as open surgery in terms of functional and oncologic outcomes and major complication rates, with the demonstrated advantages of a minimally invasive technique.

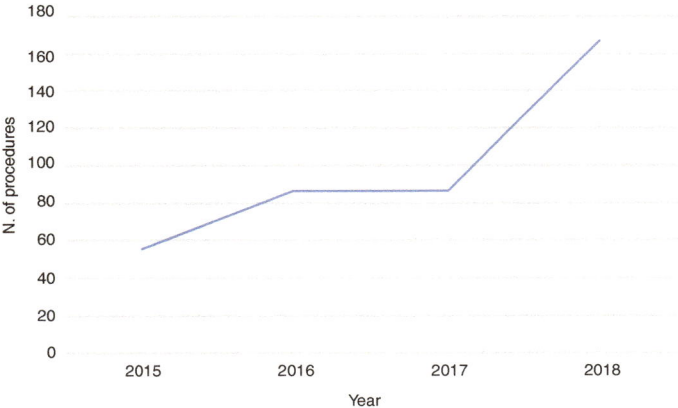

Fig. 11.1 Trend of robotic surgery for esophageal cancer in Italy 2015–2018

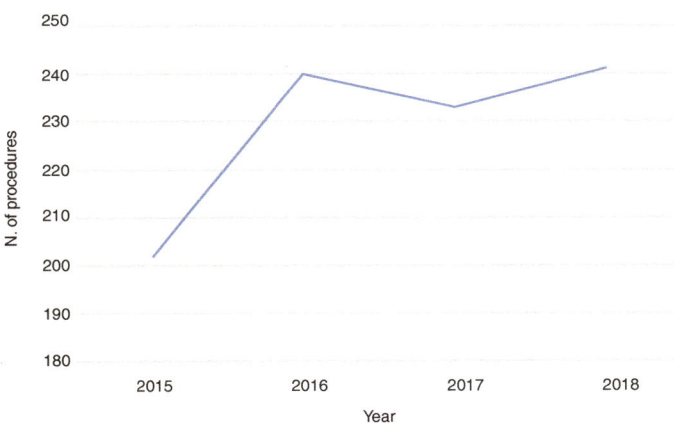

Fig. 11.2 Trend of robotic surgery for gastric cancer in Italy 2015–2018

11.2.1 Robot-Assisted Minimally Invasive Esophagectomy

Only a few studies are dedicated to the definition of the learning curve of this technically challenging operation, with some limitations due to the small number of patients included insufficient to identify the plateau, different methodology of learning curve analysis (CUSUM or arbitrarily divided groups), only McKeown or Ivor Lewis or both considered, confusion for hybrid approaches and different surgical systems used.

Twenty cases are considered by Hernandez et al. to significantly reduce the operative time of the Ivor Lewis procedure from 514 to 397 min, without variation in anastomotic leak rate; the same number of 20 is reported by Abbott et al., with a decrease in morbidity after other 10 cases [1, 2].

A significant decrease in surgical time was noted after the first 26 McKeown esophagectomies in a paper by Zhang et al. without any other difference in short-term outcomes and complications, demonstrating that the robotic approach is relatively safe even during the early experience, even though the mean number of lymph nodes harvested was greater in the second group of patients (after 26) [3].

According to the largest series of McKeown robot-assisted minimally invasive esophagectomies (RAMIE) (232 patients) described by van der Sluis et al., surgical proficiency—in terms of operative time, blood loss and conversion rate—can be achieved after 70 procedures: a reduction of the learning curve to 24 cases leads to the same results, also in terms of radicality and complications, for a second surgeon well trained and supervised by the first surgeon as a proctor [4].

In the two series including both Ivor Lewis and McKeown RAMIE, the learning curve is considered completed after respectively 30/45 and 80 cases, with a 14% decrease in overall complications in the study of Sarkaria et al. and a decrease in anastomotic leak rate from 15% to 2% in Park et al.'s series [5, 6].

These variations in terms of number of operations and time to reach the learning curve plateau is probably due to the different level of experience and volume of open and non-robotic minimally invasive esophagectomy of the team involved. The increase of morbidity during the learning period can be particularly explained in cases of need to perform a novel robotic intrathoracic anastomosis.

To reduce the risk of increasing major complications during the learning curve, Claassen et al.'s review suggested a safe implementation program based on specific guidelines, video-based platforms, training models and structured training program including proctorship. A similar approach is evident in Egberts et al.'s recommendations to develop a standardized robot-assisted Ivor Lewis surgical workflow aiming to maintain patient safety, prevent medical errors and facilitate the learning curve [7, 8].

RAMIE is a complex robotic procedure and should be reserved for experienced esophageal surgeons who are not exempted, however, from the training pathway, as they are often not very familiar with the minimally invasive techniques.

11.2.2 Robot-Assisted Gastrectomy

Most reports to date are from Eastern countries, predominantly consisting of observational studies, some of them particularly focused on the learning curve, especially compared with that of laparoscopic gastrectomy, or considering it among other topics. Also these reports suffer some limitations due to the heterogeneity of statistical methods, small and retrospective series, inclusion of distal gastrectomy alone or together with total gastrectomy, different levels of experience in open and laparoscopic gastric surgery, low body mass index (BMI), no impact estimated on oncological outcomes. Consequently, the findings should be applied with caution particularly by novel practitioners and in the Western countries where the volume of gastrectomy is lower and the stage of disease and BMI of patients are higher, with a greater proportion of total gastrectomies.

Already in 2009 Song et al., in their study comparing laparoscopic and robotic experience by a single surgeon, showed the same outcomes in terms of blood loss, hospital length of stay, oral diet and lymph node retrieval in the early phase robotic (20 cases) compared to the late phase laparoscopic (40 cases), suggesting that surgeons may more quickly become proficient with robot-assisted gastrectomy (RAG) than with laparoscopic gastrectomy [9].

In 2012 Kang et al., considering 100 cases of RAG, observed a significant difference between the first 20 cases and the subsequent 80 cases in terms of operative time and hospital length of stay; other studies [10, 11] documented shorter learning curves for RAG (11–25 procedures) compared with laparoscopic gastrectomy (40–60 procedures): these data are confirmed by Huang et al. who reported a stabilized operating time after 25 robotic operations compared to 41 in laparoscopy. Using operative time as a measure of proficiency, Harrison et al. noted a significant difference after the first 20 cases without any other correlation with length of stay and patient BMI, as instead noted in patients undergoing esophagogastrectomy [12–14].

In 2012 Park et al. analyzed the learning curve of three surgeons with different expertise in laparoscopic resection using a parametric nonlinear regression model: the stabilization of operation time for distal RAG was achieved on average after ten cases, but it was shorter and the reduction was greater for the surgeon with more laparoscopic experience. By contrast, the less experienced surgeon had more complications and his operation time was affected by patient age and BMI [15].

The findings of Kim et al. regarding the surgical success rate using the CUSUM score revealed a cut-off at the 81st case for laparoscopic surgery but no cut-off for the robotic procedure, suggesting that RAG can be performed safely from the first case if conducted by an experienced laparoscopic surgeon [16].

Subsequently Zhou et al. assessed the learning curve for two surgeons experienced in laparoscopic gastrectomy with the CUSUM score reaching the initial phase plateau at 12 and 14 cases and the mastery phase at 30 cases, but this may not reflect the real curve for non-expert surgeons: according to Nakauchi et al., a shorter learning curve for RAG may make it easier for a surgeon inexperienced in laparoscopic gastrectomy to perform RAG or for an experienced surgeon to perform complicated surgery, but this needs to be proven [17, 18].

In a similar vein, An et al. evaluated the learning curve and short-term surgical outcomes of distal RAG performed by a single surgeon experienced in open, but not laparoscopic, gastrectomy: the duration of surgery was stabilized after 25 procedures (420 min vs. 281 for the later cases). No other postoperative outcomes, including mean number of retrieved lymph nodes, differed between the two groups. Moreover, there were no conversions to open gastrectomy and postoperative complications were acceptable [19].

With the increased popularity of robotic surgery and to overcome the major limitation of a single surgeon's experience, Kim et al. very recently published the results of a multicenter prospective trial of 502 RAG specifically focused on the learning curve with a very complete statistical analysis including RA-CUSUM to depict complications during the learning curve of five surgeons already proficient in laparoscopic gastrectomy: with regard to operation time, initial proficiency was observed after about 25 cases and the plateau was reached at around 65 cases, being influenced by increased blood loss, BMI and the need for total gastrectomy. Three turning points in the RA-CUSUM curve for complications were recorded at 25, 65 and 88 identifying four phases (initial, proficiency, transitional, mastery) with 20%, 10%, 26% and 6.4% of complications, respectively: the increase in complications during the third phase (rebound phenomenon) may be due to extension of the indications and more difficult procedures, including total gastrectomy and intracorporeal anastomosis. The complication learning curve was shorter for surgeons who received mentoring and paradoxically with less experience in laparoscopic surgery, while only proctorship was unable to shorten the time to reduce complications [20].

According to these data, training in RAG is not accelerated by previous laparoscopic experience but rather by a stepwise learning curriculum starting from mentored courses with lectures, standardized laboratory training with videotape analysis, case observation and finally proctorship in the operating room.

Lastly, the above limitations due to the peculiarity of predominant Asian series suggest some caution when translating the current evidence to a European population until now involved in limited studies on RAG [21].

11.3 Robotic Pancreatic Surgery

The robotic approach to oncological pancreatic resections has progressively increased over the last decade after its feasibility and safety were acknowledged by several surgical groups worldwide [22, 23]. The known benefits of robotic technology have helped surgeons to overcome the limitations experienced during laparoscopic pancreatectomies and to recapture some of the confidence of the open approach that is essential in such a complex surgery especially for fine dissection, vascular control and anastomosis [24, 25]. A lot of recent systematic reviews and meta-analyses have attested that robotic pancreatectomies are comparable to their open equivalents in terms of short-term oncological results, morbidity and mortality rates with even better outcomes as to intraoperative blood loss, wound infection, postoperative recovery and length of hospital stay [26, 27]. However, the lack of high-quality randomized controlled trials limits the evidence of these data, which mostly come from retrospective studies performed at high-volume centers and whose results are invariably influenced by selection bias, poor standardization of techniques or unfulfilled completion of the learning curve [26]. On the other hand, recently published data obtained from national registries have shown a widespread adoption of minimally invasive pancreatectomies by low-volume centers where only a few cases per year are performed, which makes their safety and effectiveness questionable [28, 29]. Adam et al. analyzed about 1000 minimally invasive pancreaticoduodenectomies (MIPD) compared to over 6000 open cases all taken from a nationwide database and found that 92% of the hospitals performing MIPD were low-volume centers with less than ten procedures done over the 2-year observation period and that almost half of these centers had only recruited one MIPD case overall [28]. Plus, the 30-day mortality rate in this cohort was significantly higher for MIPD than for open cases [28]. The fact that the risk of postoperative death is greater when MIPD are performed at low-volume centers raises substantial concern considering that the minimally invasive approach is mostly allocated to the "easiest" patients in terms of tumor stage and comorbidities, especially at the beginning of the learning curve. The importance of hospital volume and surgeon's experience has been largely validated in the field of pancreatic cancer surgery across time regardless of the type of access used [30–32]. An inverse association between higher hospital volume and lower rates of postoperative deaths and complications as well as improved overall survival is evident in the published literature although the exact mechanism for this strong relationship is less clear [32, 33]. The individual contribution of hospital-related factors (i.e., availability of defined clinical pathways and qualified medical specialties for optimal postoperative care) rather than surgical expertise or surgeon's annual volume to this effect at high-volume centers is still debated, but it is reasonable to assume that all these elements play a key role. The rationale of this observation remains consistent even admitting that significant heterogeneity in the available data exists and that there is no agreement in the literature on the definition of high- and low-volume centers, which is often arbitrary [31]. Nevertheless, the superior quality of overall assistance and the existence of dedicated protocols for patients undergoing pancreatic resections at high-volume centers may compensate for less surgical proficiency during the learning curve. Instead, the occurrence of severe complications in resected patients at low-volume centers is likely to end up with poor prognosis as a result of the lower level of available care, even when experienced pancreatic surgeons are present [28, 33, 34]. Given the technical challenges of MIPD, the need for critical management of possible complications cannot be disregarded [23–26, 28]. Attempts made to objectively identify a minimum threshold number of MIPD to be performed yearly at high-volume centers do not fully reflect the complexity of this surgery or the time required to master the learning curve of the technique or to maintain proficiency [34]. Robotic technology is known to allow for fast achievement of surgical mastery of a given procedure and some reports have proven that increasing hands-on experience positively affects the surgical outcomes of robotic pancreatic resections [23, 24, 26, 35]; this may also translate into oncological benefits by reducing delays in the initiation of adjuvant therapies as compared to other approaches [36]. Researchers agree that prior experience with both open pancreatic resections and major laparoscopic surgery are essential for safe and effective implementation of the robotic platform in this setting [34, 37]. However, recent data confirm that minimally invasive pancreatectomies are still largely performed at low-volume centers, where these requirements are most often lacking [34].

There are several published reports supporting the so-called hub-spoke model for a rational organization of robotic surgery on a regional basis [32–34, 36, 37]. Such an organizational network implies an elevated integration between the provider of robotic procedures (hub) and other institutions (spokes), which results in several advantages for patients, professionals, and the healthcare system. This model fully complies with the mindset of optimizing the effectiveness of robotic surgery while minimizing the risks and limiting the costs. Provided that hospital volume is an independent and critical factor for the outcomes of major oncological surgery, it is clear that only a high-volume center embodies the hub to which pancreatic cancer cases suitable for the robotic approach should be directed [28, 31–34, 37]: this is where adequate training and skill set have been acquired, structured pathways for postoperative care are established and the available resources, both human and instrumental, allow for successful outcomes of these complex though safe procedures in experienced hands [28, 31, 34, 37]. In a social and economic perspective, the investment of healthcare providers to support robotic pancreas programs in a regional or national network may be offset by the patients' faster return to productiveness and fewer long-term consequences related to large wound abdominal surgery [35].

11.4   Robotic Colorectal Surgery

Robotic surgery represents a further step forward in the evolution of minimally invasive surgery and one of the major innovations in the surgical field of the last decades from a technological standpoint. The perceived advantages of robotic surgery, including ergonomics and the ability to operate in the confined anatomic space of the pelvis, have made proctectomy for rectal cancer a particularly attractive target for robotic surgery. As a result, since the first published reports of robotic colectomies in 2002, a large number of colorectal procedures have been performed with robotic assistance [38–40].

All new surgical techniques and innovations need a learning curve, with accumulating experience being associated with improved outcomes [41]. Surgeon experience is usually evaluated based on annual volume and the best early postoperative surgical outcomes are achieved in centers where there are high cumulative and high annual volume surgeons [42].

11.4.1 Hospital and Surgeon Volume: An Update

Keller et al. evaluated the outcomes of robotic colorectal procedures in the setting of different surgeon and hospital volumes. A United States inpatient database (NIS) was reviewed for robotic colorectal resections performed during an 18-month period. Hospitals and surgeons were stratified into high, average, and low case volumes based on a normal distribution scale. High, average, and low volume was defined as ≤10, 11 to 20, and >20, respectively, for hospitals, and ≤5, 6–15, and >15, respectively, for surgeons. Short-term outcomes and hospital cost were evaluated. Low volume was associated with significantly higher overall complication rates, longer length of stay and higher costs [43]. A more recent study compared oncologic outcomes with center-level robotic rectal resection volume. More than

8000 patients with rectal adenocarcinoma who underwent robotic rectal resection were identified in the United States National Cancer Database. On multivariate regression analysis, lower center-level volume of robotic rectal resection was associated with significantly higher rates of conversion to open, positive margins, inadequate lymph node harvest (≥ 12), and lower overall survival [44].

A case sequence analysis recently reported improved outcomes with increasing cumulative experience. After completing 27 cases of robotic colorectal resection, a reduction in iatrogenic complications was noted, and this trend continued as volume increased [45].

The main concern about these studies is the retrospective analysis performed, evaluating data derived from administrative database, but probably these studies are more adherent to real life.

11.4.2 Complication Rates in Robotic Colorectal Surgery

The largest randomized control trial published on robotic rectal resection compared to laparoscopic rectal surgery (ROLARR trial) did not demonstrate an increase in complication rates in the robotic arm. Furthermore, the surgeons participating to the trial were still in the learning curve phase for robotic rectal resection, and their results in term of conversion rates improved with the increasing number of robotic rectal procedures performed [46].

On the other hand, several studies have demonstrated a reduction in postoperative complications for robotic surgical procedures, when compared to conventional open or laparoscopic surgery [47–49].

An ACS NSQUIP nationwide database analysis including patients subjected to low anterior rectal resection has recently shown a statistically significant reduction in overall septic complication rates and surgical site infection rates (1.6% in robotic vs. 3.1% in laparoscopic procedures, $p = 0.02$). Bivariate analysis and logistic regression models were used [49].

Different studies have shown a reduction in conversion rates of robotic colorectal surgery when compared to conventional laparoscopy. Sun et al. analyzed data from the US National cancer database including 6000 patients and demonstrated a reduction in conversion rates (8% vs. 16%, $p < 0.001$) in favor of the robotic group. It is worth underlining that in the robotic group a higher number of male patients subjected to preoperative radio-chemotherapy for locally advanced rectal cancer (cT3N+) was recorded; these factors are well-known predictors of technical procedural complexity [50].

Similar results regarding robotic versus laparoscopic low anterior resection were reported by other US population-based studies from the ACS NSQIP database and Michigan Surgical Quality Collaborative Registry carried out between 2012 and 2014 [49, 51]. Reduction in complications and conversion to open surgery can conceptually and potentially reduce the length of hospital stay, thereby reducing the overall indirect costs related to hospitalization and the possible subsequent need for outpatient visits, with a return to normal daily activity and practice. The ACS NSQIP study including more than 11,000 patients supports this finding, having demonstrated a reduction in postoperative length of stay for patients subjected to robotic versus laparoscopic rectal resection (4.5 vs. 5.3 days, $p < 0.001$) [49].

The Michigan Surgical Quality Collaborative Registry, including patients subjected to minimally invasive colorectal resection (from 2012 to 2014) further corroborates the above data and tried to specifically focus on the relationship between reduction in complication/conversion rates and costs. In this case, the total episode cost (namely in-hospital direct costs plus 30-day post-discharge overall costs) was considered: total costs were comparable in the robotic and laparoscopic group, with the lower conversion rates of robotic surgery (and subsequent reduction in complications and length of stay) balancing the higher direct costs related to instrumentation and operating room occupation time [51].

Salman et al. also showed similar results. When the overall cost is considered, hospitalization cost involving robotic surgery appears to be cheaper than its laparoscopic and open counterparts, because of lower complication rates, less intensive care unit stay and shorter length of stay [52].

Better clinical outcomes in robotic colorectal surgery are probably related to the concept of "precision surgery" in robotics, which allows for a reduction in tissue trauma through a more precise exposure and dissection along embryological planes, thus also reducing intraoperative blood loss.

11.4.3 Training in Robotic Colorectal Surgery

The learning curve and adequate training in robotic surgery have a crucial role in reducing complication rates. The planning of a structured training program is fundamental to flatten the learning curve and speed up the process of optimizing both short- and long-term surgical outcomes. We have demonstrated the safety and efficacy of a structured training program for young novice surgeons without prior experience in both open and laparoscopic colorectal surgery, who were autonomous in basic minimally invasive surgical procedures. Right colectomy with intracorporeal anastomosis was chosen as a model and divided into three main learning modules (colonic mobilization, vascular control, intracorporeal anastomosis). Each step was carried out by the trainees at least twice under direct supervision of the senior surgeon. After the initial robotic cases performed completely under formal proctoring, the trainees went on to perform robotic right colectomy independently without a mentor, for a total of 20 procedures. This structured stepwise approach allowed junior surgeons to safely and effectively perform right colectomies with intracorporeal anastomosis. Neither conversion to open surgery nor intraoperative or major postoperative complications were recorded, thus allowing the novice to achieve results comparable to the senior surgeon's case series [53].

To summarize, even in robotic colorectal surgery the effect of the learning curve, case volume and surgeon volume are strictly related to clinical and oncologic outcomes. It is fundamental to carefully evaluate hospital and single-surgeon volumes and to plan a structured training program before adopting a new technology like robotic surgery.

References

1. Hernandez JM, Dimou F, Weber J, et al. Defining the learning curve for robotic-assisted esophagogastrectomy. J Gastrointest Surg. 2013;17(8):1346–51.
2. Abbott A, Shridhar R, Hoffe S, et al. Robotic assisted Ivor Lewis esophagectomy in the elderly patient. J Gastrointest Oncol. 2015;6(1):31–8.
3. Zhang H, Chen L, Wang Z, et al. The learning curve for robotic McKeown esophagectomy in patients with esophageal cancer. Ann Thorac Surg. 2018;105(4):1024–30.
4. van der Sluis PC, Ruurda JP, van der Horst S, et al. Learning curve for robot-assisted minimally invasive thoracoscopic esophagectomy: results from 312 cases. Ann Thorac Surg. 2018;106(1):264–71.
5. Sarkaria IS, Rizk NP, Grosser R, et al. Attaining proficiency in robotic-assisted minimally invasive esophagectomy while maximizing safety during procedure development. Innovations (Phila). 2016;11(4):268–73.
6. Park S, Hyun K, Lee HJ, et al. A study of the learning curve for robotic oesophagectomy for oesophageal cancer. Eur J Cardiothorac Surg. 2018;53(4):862–70.
7. Claassen L, van Workum F, Rosman C. Learning curve and postoperative outcomes of minimally invasive esophagectomy. J Thorac Dis. 2019;11(Suppl 5):S777–85.
8. Egberts J-H, Biebl M, Perez DR, et al. Robot-assisted oesophagectomy: recommendations towards a standardised Ivor Lewis procedure. J Gastrointest Surg. 2019;23(7):1485–92.
9. Song J, Kang WH, Oh SJ, et al. Role of robotic gastrectomy using da Vinci system compared with laparoscopic gastrectomy: initial experience of 20 consecutive cases. Surg Endosc. 2009;23(6):1204–11.
10. Son T, Hyung WJ. Robotic gastrectomy for gastric cancer. J Surg Oncol. 2015;112(3):271–8.
11. Suda K, Nakauchi M, Inaba K, et al. Minimally invasive surgery for upper gastrointestinal cancer: our experience and review of the literature. World J Gastroenterol. 2016;22(19):4626–37.
12. Kang BH, Xuan Y, Hur H, et al. Comparison of surgical outcomes between robotic and laparoscopic gastrectomy for gastric cancer: the learning curve of robotic surgery. J Gastric Cancer. 2012;12(3):156–63.
13. Huang K-H, Lan Y-T, Fang W-L, et al. Comparison of the operative outcomes and learning curves between laparoscopic and robotic gastrectomy for gastric cancer. PLoS One. 2014;9(10):e111499. https://doi.org/10.1371/journal.pone.0111499.
14. Harrison LE, Yiengpruksawan A, Patel J, et al. Robotic gastrectomy and esophagogastrectomy: a single center experience of 105 cases. J Surg Oncol. 2015;112(8):888–93.
15. Park S-S, Kim M-C, Park MS, Hyung WJ. Rapid adaptation of robotic gastrectomy for gastric cancer by experienced laparoscopic surgeons. Surg Endosc. 2012;26(1):60–7.
16. Kim H-I, Park MS, Song KJ, et al. Rapid and safe learning of robotic gastrectomy for gastric cancer: multidimensional analysis in a comparison with laparoscopic gastrectomy. Eur J Surg Oncol. 2014;40(10):1346–54.
17. Zhou J, Shi Y, Qian F, et al. Cumulative summation analysis of learning curve for robot-assisted gastrectomy in gastric cancer. J Surg Oncol. 2015;111(6):760–7.
18. Nakauchi M, Uyama I, Suda K, et al. Robotic surgery for the upper gastrointestinal tract: current status and future perspectives. Asian J Endosc Surg. 2017;10(4):354–63.
19. An JY, Kim SM, Ahn S, et al. Successful robotic gastrectomy does not require extensive laparoscopic experience. J Gastric Cancer. 2018;18(1):90–8.
20. Kim MS, Kim WJ, Hyung WJ, et al. Comprehensive learning curve of robotic surgery: discovery from a multicenter prospective trial of robotic gastrectomy. Ann Surg. 2019. https://doi.org/10.1097/SLA.0000000000003583. [Epub ahead of print].

21. van Boxel GI, Ruurda JP, van Hillegersberg R. Robotic-assisted gastrectomy for gastric cancer: a European perspective. Gastric Cancer. 2019;22(5):909–19.
22. Giulianotti PC, Sbrana F, Bianco FM, et al. Robot-assisted laparoscopic pancreatic surgery: single-surgeon experience. Surg Endosc. 2010;24(7):1646–57.
23. Zureikat AH, Moser AJ, Boone BA, et al. 250 robotic pancreatic resections: safety and feasibility. Ann Surg. 2013;258:554–9; discussion 559–62.
24. Boggi U, Napoli N, Costa F, et al. Robotic-assisted pancreatic resections. World J Surg. 2016;40(10):2497–506.
25. Xourafas D, Ashley SW, Clancy TE. Comparison of perioperative outcomes between open, laparoscopic and robotic distal pancreatectomy: an analysis of 1815 patients from the ACS-NSQIP procedure-targeted pancreatectomy database. J Gastrointest Surg. 2017;21(9):1442–52.
26. Zhao W, Liu C, Li S, et al. Safety and efficacy for robot-assisted versus open pancreaticoduodenectomy and distal pancreatectomy: a systematic review and meta-analysis. Surg Oncol. 2018;27(3):468–78.
27. McMillan MT, Zureikat AH, Hogg ME, et al. A propensity score-matched analysis of robotic vs open pancreaticoduodenectomy on incidence of pancreatic fistula. JAMA Surg. 2017;152(4):327–35.
28. Adam MA, Choudhury K, Dinan MA, et al. Minimally invasive versus open pancreaticoduodenectomy for cancer: practice patterns and short-term outcomes among 7061 patients. Ann Surg. 2015;262(2):372–7.
29. Sharpe SM, Talamonti MS, Wang CE, et al. Early national experience with laparoscopic pancreaticoduodenectomy for ductal adenocarcinoma: a comparison of laparoscopic pancreaticoduodenectomy and open pancreaticoduodenectomy from the National Cancer Data Base. J Am Coll Surg. 2015;221(1):175–84.
30. Lieberman MD, Kilburn H, Lindsey M, Brennan MF. Relation of perioperative deaths to hospital volume among patients undergoing pancreatic resection for malignancy. Ann Surg. 1995;222(5):638–45.
31. Hata T, Motoi F, Ishida M, et al. Effect of hospital volume on surgical outcomes after pancreaticoduodenectomy: a systematic review and meta-analysis. Ann Surg. 2016;263(4):664–72.
32. Gooiker GA, van Gijn W, Wouters MW, et al.; Signalling Committee Cancer of the Dutch Cancer Society. Systematic review and meta-analysis of the volume-outcome relationship in pancreatic surgery. Br J Surg. 2011;98(4):485–94.
33. Schmidt CM, Turrini O, Parikh P, et al. Effect of hospital volume, surgeon experience, and surgeon volume on patient outcomes after pancreaticoduodenectomy: a single-institution experience. Arch Surg. 2010;145(7):634–40.
34. Adam MA, Thomas S, Youngwirth L, et al. Defining a hospital volume threshold for minimally invasive pancreaticoduodenectomy in the United States. JAMA Surg. 2017;152(4):336–42.
35. Stafford AT, Walsh RM. Robotic surgery of the pancreas: the current state of the art. J Surg Oncol. 2015;112(3):289–94.
36. Wright GP, Zureikat AH. Development of minimally invasive pancreatic surgery: an evidence-based systematic review of laparoscopic versus robotic approaches. J Gastrointest Surg. 2016;20(9):1658–65.
37. Nota CL, Zwart MJ, Fong Y, et al. Developing a robotic pancreas program: the Dutch experience. J Vis Surg. 2017;3:106. https://doi.org/10.21037/jovs.2017.07.02.
38. Marcus HJ, Hughes-Hallett A, Payne CJ, et al. Trends in the diffusion of robotic surgery: a retrospective observational study. Int J Med Robot. 2017;13(4):e1870. https://doi.org/10.1002/rcs.1870.
39. Delaney CP, Lynch AC, Senagore AJ, Fazio VW. Comparison of robotically performed and traditional laparoscopic colorectal surgery. Dis Colon Rectum. 2003;46(12):1633–9.
40. Bianchi PP, Luca F, Petz W, et al. The role of the robotic technique in minimally invasive surgery in rectal cancer. Ecancermedicalscience. 2013;7:357. https://doi.org/10.3332/ecancer.2013.357.
41. Jiménez-Rodríguez RM, Rubio-Dorado-Manzanares M, Díaz-Pavón JM, et al. Learning curve in robotic rectal cancer surgery: current state of affairs. Int J Color Dis. 2016;31(12):1807–15.

42. Yeo HL, Abelson JS, Mao J, et al. Surgeon annual and cumulative volumes predict early post-operative outcomes after rectal cancer resection. Ann Surg. 2017;265(1):151–7.
43. Keller DS, Hashemi L, Lu M, Delaney CP. Short-term outcomes for robotic colorectal surgery by provider volume. J Am Coll Surg. 2013;217(6):1063–9.e1.
44. Concors SJ, Murken DR, Hernandez PT, et al. The volume-outcome relationship in robotic proctectomy: does center volume matter? Results of a national cohort study. Surg Endosc. 2019. https://doi.org/10.1007/s00464-019-07227-6. [Epub ahead of print].
45. Symer MM, Sedrakyan A, Yeo HL. Case sequence analysis of the robotic colorectal resection learning curve. Dis Colon Rectum. 2019;62(9):1071–8.
46. Jayne D, Pigazzi A, Marshall H, et al. Effect of robotic-assisted vs conventional laparoscopic surgery on risk of conversion to open laparotomy among patients undergoing resection for rectal cancer: the ROLARR randomized clinical trial. JAMA. 2017;318:1569–80.
47. Liu CA, Huang KH, Chen MH, et al. Comparison of the surgical outcomes of minimally invasive and open surgery for octogenarian and older compared to younger gastric cancer patients: a retrospective cohort study. BMC Surg. 2017;17(1):68. https://doi.org/10.1186/s12893-017-0265-3.
48. Plotkin A, Ceppa EP, Zarzaur BL, et al. Reduced morbidity with minimally invasive distal pancreatectomy for pancreatic adenocarcinoma. HPB (Oxford). 2017;19(3):279–85.
49. Bhama AR, Obias V, Welch KB, et al. A comparison of laparoscopic and robotic colorectal surgery outcomes using the American College of Surgeons National Surgical Quality Improvement Program (ACS NSQIP) database. Surg Endosc. 2016;30(4):1576–84.
50. Sun Z, Kim J, Adam MA, et al. Minimally invasive versus open low anterior resection: equivalent survival in a national analysis of 14,033 patients with rectal cancer. Ann Surg. 2016;263(6):1152–8.
51. Cleary RK, Mullard AJ, Ferraro J, Regenbogen SE. The cost of conversion in robotic and laparoscopic colorectal surgery. Surg Endosc. 2018;32(3):1515–24.
52. Salman M, Bell T, Martin J, et al. Use, cost, complications, and mortality of robotic versus nonrobotic general surgery procedures based on a nationwide database. Am Surg. 2013;79(6):553–60.
53. Formisano G, Esposito S, Coratti F, et al. Structured training program in colorectal surgery: the robotic surgeon as a new paradigm. Minerva Chir. 2018;74(2):17–5.

The Specific Role of Minimally Invasive Robotic Endocrine Surgery

12

Micaela Piccoli, Sofia Esposito, and Barbara Mullineris

12.1 Thyroid and Parathyroid Robotic Surgery

Although the first report of an endoscopic neck procedure was in 1996 [1], minimally invasive procedures in head and neck surgery have not been widely adopted, owing to limitations associated with the anatomy of the neck, such as the narrow field, limited working space, and contiguity of critical vessels and nerves. Robotic surgery may overcome some of the well-known limitations of endoscopy, such as collisions and limited range of motion of the rigid instruments, unstable vision, two-dimensional image, and uncomfortable ergonomics. The robotic system provides enhanced visualization with the three-dimensional view of the surgical field, tremor filtering and improved instrument range of motion. These characteristics offer several advantages for the surgeon, especially in confined areas like the neck and mediastinum, allowing finer dissection and better control of the instruments. Since the first report of a transaxillary robot-assisted gasless thyroidectomy by Kang et al. [2], several studies have confirmed the feasibility and safety of robotic thyroidectomy and parathyroidectomy in selected patients [3–8].

The robotic approach has been reported to have a shorter learning curve compared with conventional endoscopic techniques. Lee et al. demonstrated the superiority of robotic thyroidectomy compared to the endoscopic technique in terms of operative time, lymph node dissection, and learning curve. The learning curve for robotic thyroidectomy was reported to be 35–40 cases, in contrast to 55–60 cases for endoscopic thyroidectomy [9]. Kandil et al. also confirmed a learning curve of 45 cases, highlighting the technical challenges to be expected in obese patients [8].

Nevertheless, this approach was welcomed with criticism, especially in the United States. American surgeons questioned the transferability of the Korean

M. Piccoli (✉) · S. Esposito · B. Mullineris
Division of General, Emergency Surgery and New Technologies,
Baggiovara General Hospital, Modena, Italy
e-mail: piccoli.micaela@aou.mo.it; esposito.sofia@aou.mo.it; mullineris.barbara@aou.mo.it

© Springer Nature Switzerland AG 2021
M. Montorsi (ed.), *Volume-Outcome Relationship in Oncological Surgery*,
Updates in Surgery, https://doi.org/10.1007/978-3-030-51806-6_12

experience to the Western population in view of differences in patient character-istics and nature of the disease [10]. Koreans have a higher incidence of sub-centimeter nodules, smaller body size, and smaller thyroidectomy resections (average volume resected in the United States is double that in Korea) [11]. In response to these statements, Western surgeons performing robotic thyroidecto-mies in high-volume centers demonstrated that, with minimal modifications in patient arm positioning, this technique could be implemented in their patient populations, without significantly increasing operative time or complications [4, 8, 12].

Another reason for skepticism is also represented by the high costs related to robotic surgery. Cabot et al. compared standard cervical thyroidectomy with con-ventional transaxillary endoscopic and transaxillary robotic thyroidectomy. Although a higher total cost for the transaxillary approaches was reported, a signifi-cant decrease in transaxillary operative times resulted in cost equivalence between the techniques. They also stated that increasing the yearly load decreases the cost of transaxillary robotic and endoscopic thyroidectomy, but not to the point of cost equivalence with the standard cervical technique [13].

Robotic parathyroidectomy is even less widespread as a result of the presence of several minimal access techniques, in which the parathyroid procedure is performed with a small neck incision (less than 2.5 cm), which have proved to be safe and cost-effective [14]. To date, only few non-randomized studies have compared the out-comes of robotic parathyroidectomy with targeted minimally invasive parathyroidectomy (MIP). Most authors concluded that robotic parathyroidectomy is a feasible and safe alternative to MIP, but improved cosmesis should be weighed against longer operative times and higher costs [15–17]. However, the robotic trans-axillary approach represents a valid alternative for patients with mediastinal para-thyroid adenomas, as reported by several institutions [18, 19]. Mediastinal adenomas in 1/3 of the cases cannot be reached cervically and require a sternotomy or thora-cotomy, with increased morbidity. Robotic parathyroidectomy not only offers cos-metic benefits due to the single skin incision in a neutral area but it also results in faster return to functional activities, less pain and morbidity, when compared to the transthoracic approach [6, 18, 19].

In the United States, from 2009 through early 2011, there was a steady increase in the volume of robotic thyroidectomies, especially among high-volume institu-tions [20]. In October 2011, Intuitive Surgical (Sunnyvale, CA) sent a notice with-drawing its support to robotic thyroid surgery. This caused a drop in robotic thyroidectomy volumes and a transition of the procedure to low-volume centers (fewer than five cases annually). In their recent study, Hinson et al. reported that low-volume centers had higher complication rates when compared to high-volume institutions, but they were also responsible for the majority of the robotic thyroidec-tomy performed in the United States [20].

In 2016, the American Thyroid Association stated that remote-access robotic thyroidectomy had proven to be safe and feasible in high-volume centers and had a role in selected circumstances. Patients for whom avoidance of a neck incision is of utmost value, because of either cosmetic or wound healing issues, should see their wishes acknowledged and fulfilled, as long as the procedure is done by experienced surgeons under strict selection criteria [21].

Surgeon volume has always been considered an important predictor of clinical and economic outcomes in conventional open endocrine surgery. Surgeons performing fewer than four endocrine operations yearly are responsible for disproportionately high complication rates, while surgeons performing 100 procedures maintain the lowest complication rates [22]. Robotic-assisted remote-access neck surgery requires an additional level of expertise of the surgeon and the institution. This approach necessitates dedicated tools (specific retractor, 5 mm robotic instruments) as well as a specialized surgical and operating room team.

Considering that robotic thyroidectomy requires approximately 40 cases to become proficient [23] and higher-volume centers have significantly lower complication rates, centralization of volume into higher-volume centers could be beneficial for patients, while decentralization may be associated with increased complication rates [20]; high-volume centers could also have an advantage in terms of cost-effectiveness, with shorter operative time, shorter hospital stay and better deployment of resources [13].

12.2   Adrenal Gland Robotic Surgery

Laparoscopic adrenalectomy is considered to be the gold standard treatment for benign adrenal diseases. Malignancy and large tumors are still considered a contraindication to the minimally invasive approach. The robotic platform has found its use also in adrenal surgery, proving to be a safe and feasible alternative to laparoscopy [24]. Both posterior retroperitoneal and lateral transabdominal approach techniques have proved to be safe and feasible with the robotic system [25]. Literature reports regarding robotic adrenalectomy have significantly increased in number in the last decade, but we are still lacking high-quality trials in terms of evidence-based medicine. Compared to conventional laparoscopic surgery, the current literature indicates an advantage in intraoperative blood loss and length of hospital stay, with similar morbidity and operative times [24, 26].

The robotic platform, with its intrinsic characteristics such as tremor filtering, enhanced 3D vision, and instruments with a wider range of motion, provides a substantial advantage when precise dissection in narrow surgical fields is required, thus potentially reducing the learning curve. Brunaud et al. reported a learning curve of 20 cases, with independent predictors of operative time being surgeon experience, first assistant training level, and tumor size [27].

The robotic platform could offer an advantage also in large tumors. Agcaoglu et al. compared robotic and laparoscopic adrenalectomy for tumors larger than 5 cm and found that operative time, conversion rate and length of hospital stay were shorter in the robotic group [16]. In their recent study, Quadri et al. reported that patient BMI, tumor side and size did not have a negative impact on perioperative and postoperative outcomes of robotic adrenalectomy, concluding that the robotic platform could have an impact on expanding the indications of minimally invasive surgery.

The main criticism toward robotic surgery remains cost-effectiveness [28]. Brunaud et al. also analyzed costs related to robotic adrenalectomy and found that the robotic procedure was 2.3 times more costly than lateral transperitoneal laparoscopic adrenalectomy. This difference would become smaller if the number of cases per year of robotic adrenalectomy increased [27]. Recently, Feng et al. compared 58 robotic and 64 laparoscopic adrenalectomies, reporting similar anesthesia and procedure times for both procedures. Moreover, the authors demonstrated that an experienced surgical team can keep the costs of robotics comparable to those of conventional laparoscopy by limiting the number of robotic instruments and energy devices [29].

Number of cases per year is an important factor that not only influences cost-effectiveness, but mainly impacts postoperative morbidity and length of hospital stay. A recent national-level analysis of 6712 patients who underwent adrenalectomy between 1998 and 2009 demonstrated that increased surgeon volume was associated with better outcomes. The authors also identified a surgeon volume threshold of six or more procedures per year that was related with improved outcomes and decreased hospital cost [30]. Another study by Palazzo et al. also chose a threshold of six procedures per year to define high-volume surgeons. The authors used the Hospital Episode Statistics data from the National Health Service in England and demonstrated that low-volume surgeons had longer length of hospital stay and higher 30-day-readmission rates [31].

Recently, the European Society of Endocrine Surgeons (ESES) published a consensus statement on volume-outcome correlation in adrenal surgery and stated that adrenal surgery should continue only in centers performing at least six cases per year, while surgery for adrenocortical cancer should be restricted to centers performing at least 12 adrenal operations per year, underlining the importance of an integrated multidisciplinary team. Furthermore, recommendations regarding specifically robotic adrenalectomy were made. The panel stated that "robotic adrenal surgery should be implemented only in units with previous experience in robotic surgery, familiar with laparoscopic adrenalectomy and with large-volume practice. Robotic adrenalectomy is not a technique for the occasional adrenal surgeon with minimal previous personal experience (level of evidence V/grade of recommendation C)." [32].

This statement further supports the need for an organized planning of the resources in robotic surgery due to high costs of the technology and the requirement of specific expertise, as suggested also by the Health Technologies Assessment Report of the Italian Health Ministry [33].

References

1. Gagner M. Endoscopic subtotal parathyroidectomy in patients with primary hyperparathyroidism. Br J Surg. 1996;83(6):875. https://doi.org/10.1002/bjs.1800830656.
2. Kang S-W, Lee SC, Lee SH, et al. Robotic thyroid surgery using a gasless, transaxillary approach and the da Vinci S system: the operative outcomes of 338 consecutive patients. Surgery. 2009;146(6):1048–55.

3. Piccoli M, Mullineris B, Santi D, Gozzo D. Advances in robotic transaxillary thyroidectomy in Europe. Curr Surg Rep. 2017;5(8):17. https://doi.org/10.1007/s40137-017-0180-7.
4. Al Kadah B, Piccoli M, Mullineris B, et al. Modifications of transaxillary approach in endoscopic da Vinci-assisted thyroid and parathyroid gland surgery. J Robot Surg. 2015;9(1):37–44.
5. Piccoli M, Mullineris B, Gozzo D, et al. Evolution strategies in transaxillary robotic thyroidectomy: considerations on the first 449 cases performed. J Laparoendosc Adv Surg Tech. 2019;29(4):433–40.
6. Taskin HE, Arslan NC, Aliyev S, Berber E. Robotic endocrine surgery: state of the art. World J Surg. 2013;37(12):2731–9.
7. Giulianotti PC, Addeo P, Buchs NC, et al. Robotic thyroidectomy: an initial experience with the gasless transaxillary approach. J Laparoendosc Adv Surg Tech. 2012;22(4):387–91.
8. Kandil EH, Noureldine SI, Yao L, Slakey DP. Robotic transaxillary thyroidectomy: an examination of the first one hundred cases. J Am Coll Surg. 2012;214(4):558–64; discussion 564–6.
9. Lee J, Yun JH, Choi UJ, et al. Robotic versus endoscopic thyroidectomy for thyroid cancers: a multi-institutional analysis of early postoperative outcomes and surgical learning curves. J Oncol. 2012;2012:734541. https://doi.org/10.1155/2012/734541.
10. Inabnet WB III. Robotic thyroidectomy: must we drive a luxury sedan to arrive at our destination safely? Thyroid. 2012;22(10):988–90.
11. Lin H-S, Folbe AJ, Carron MA, et al. Single-incision transaxillary robotic thyroidectomy: challenges and limitations in a North American population. Otolaryngol Head Neck Surg. 2012;147(6):1041–6.
12. Kuppersmith RB, Holsinger FC. Robotic thyroid surgery: an initial experience with North American patients. Laryngoscope. 2011;121(3):521–6.
13. Cabot JC, Lee CR, Brunaud L, et al. Robotic and endoscopic transaxillary thyroidectomies may be cost prohibitive when compared to standard cervical thyroidectomy: a cost analysis. Surgery. 2012;152(6):1016–24.
14. Palazzo FF, Delbridge LW. Minimal-access/minimally invasive parathyroidectomy for primary hyperparathyroidism. Surg Clin North Am. 2004;84(3):717–34.
15. Liu SY, Lang BH. Revisiting robotic approaches to endocrine neoplasia: do the data support their continued use? Curr Opin Oncol. 2016;28(1):26–36.
16. Foley CS, Agcaoglu O, Siperstein AE, Berber E. Robotic transaxillary endocrine surgery: a comparison with conventional open technique. Surg Endosc. 2012;26(8):2259–66.
17. Noureldine SI, Lewing N, Tufano RP, Kandil E. The role of the robotic-assisted transaxillary gasless approach for the removal of parathyroid adenomas. ORL J Otorhinolaryngol Relat Spec. 2014;76(1):19–24.
18. Gonzalez-Ciccarelli LF, Esposito S, Bevere A, Giulianotti PC. Robotic transaxillary parathyroidectomy for upper mediastinal parathyroid adenoma: a case report. JSM Clin Case Rep. 2016;4(3):1107. https://www.jscimedcentral.com/CaseReports/casereports-4-1107.pdf.
19. Harvey A, Bohacek L, Neumann D, et al. Robotic thoracoscopic mediastinal parathyroidectomy for persistent hyperparathyroidism: case report and review of the literature. Surg Laparosc Endosc Percutan Tech. 2011;21(1):e24–7.
20. Hinson AM, Kandil E, O'Brien S, et al. Trends in robotic thyroid surgery in the United States from 2009 through 2013. Thyroid. 2015;25(8):919–26.
21. Berber E, Bernet V, Fahey TJ, et al. American thyroid association statement on remote-access thyroid surgery. Thyroid. 2016;26(3):331–7.
22. Stavrakis AI, Ituarte PHG, Ko CY, Yeh MW. Surgeon volume as a predictor of outcomes in inpatient and outpatient endocrine surgery. Surgery. 2007;142(6):887–99.
23. Zaidi N, Daskalaki D, Quadri P, et al. The current status of robotic transaxillary thyroidectomy in the United States: an experience from two centers. Gland Surg. 2017;6(4):380–4.
24. Makay O, Erol V, Ozdemir M. Robotic adrenalectomy. Gland Surg. 2019;8(Suppl 1):S10–6.
25. Kahramangil B, Berber E. Comparison of posterior retroperitoneal and transabdominal lateral approaches in robotic adrenalectomy: an analysis of 200 cases. Surg Endosc. 2018;32(4):1984–9.

26. Agrusa A, Romano G, Navarra G, et al. Innovation in endocrine surgery: robotic versus laparoscopic adrenalectomy. Meta-analysis and systematic literature review. Oncotarget. 2017;8(6):102392–400.
27. Brunaud L, Ayav A, Zarnegar R, et al. Prospective evaluation of 100 robotic-assisted unilateral adrenalectomies. Surgery. 2008;144(6):995–1001.
28. Quadri P, Esposito S, Coleoglou A, et al. Robotic adrenalectomy: are we expanding the indications of minimally invasive surgery? J Laparoendosc Adv Surg Tech. 2019;29(1):19–23.
29. Feng Z, Feng MP, Feng DP, et al. A cost-conscious approach to robotic adrenalectomy. J Robot Surg. 2018;12(4):607–11.
30. Anderson KL, Thomas SM, Adam MA, et al. Each procedure matters: threshold for surgeon volume to minimize complications and decrease cost associated with adrenalectomy. Surgery. 2018;163(1):157–64.
31. Palazzo F, Dickinson A, Phillips B, et al. Adrenal surgery in England: better outcomes in high-volume practices. Clin Endocrinol. 2016;85(1):17–20.
32. Mihai R, Donatini G, Vidal O, Brunaud L. Volume-outcome correlation in adrenal surgery—an ESES consensus statement. Langenbeck's Arch Surg. 2019;404(7):795–806.
33. Jefferson TO, Abraha J, Chiarolla E, et al. Chirurgia robotica, Roma. 2017. https://www.sifoweb.it/images/news-allegati/C_17_pagineAree_1202_listaFile_itemName_15_file.pdf.

Combining Risk Management and Real Time Indicator Monitoring for Continuous Improvement

13

Marco Albini, Patrizia Meroni, and Marco Montorsi

13.1 Clinical Governance and Risk Management

In 2004, Som defined clinical governance as a "governance system for health-care organizations that promotes an integrated approach towards management of inputs, structures and process to improve the outcome of health-care service delivery where health staff work in an environment of greater accountability for clinical quality" [1]. Numerous elements are necessary for the application of clinical governance. As presented by Gottwald and Lansdown in 2014 [2], these components included: research and development, evidence-based practice education and training, risk management, audit, and complaints.

In particular, risk management and audits are key components in delivering clinical governance due to the high risks present in healthcare settings and the need to assess and mitigate these risks. The importance of these two factors arose from events revealing lack of clinical safety, such as the Bristol Royal Infirmary case (inquiry started in 1991) [3], and publications highlighting the prevalence of medical errors, such as to "To err is Human" in 2000 [4]. The realization of the need for clinical safety led to a movement devoted to reducing risk and building healthcare quality assessment methods and tools [5, 6]. Indeed, over the last three decades

M. Albini (✉)
Quality Monitoring Office, Humanitas Clinical and Research Center IRCCS,
Rozzano, Milan, Italy
e-mail: marco.albini@humanitas.it

P. Meroni
Quality Management, Humanitas Clinical and Research Center IRCCS, Rozzano, Milan, Italy
e-mail: patrizia.meroni@humanitas.it

M. Montorsi
Department of Biomedical Sciences, Humanitas University, Pieve Emanuele, Milan, Italy
Department of General Surgery, Humanitas Clinical and Research Center IRCCS, Rozzano, Milan, Italy
e-mail: marco.montorsi@hunimed.eu

© Springer Nature Switzerland AG 2021
M. Montorsi (ed.), *Volume-Outcome Relationship in Oncological Surgery*,
Updates in Surgery, https://doi.org/10.1007/978-3-030-51806-6_13

many institutions have developed systems that are able to detect and gather event-related information to evaluate the risks involved in an incident, conduct present-day risk assessments and set in place appropriate mitigation strategies. Such systems are linked to a higher incident reporting that trigger improved hospital risk management activities [7]. Surgical practices have also become involved with clinical governance and risk management, as seen in numerous scenarios [8], assisting surgeons in refining their procedures and acquiring a self-improvement mindset [9].

The potential of improving healthcare service delivery relies on the possibility of detecting faults and preventing possible complications. However, considering the increasing number of healthcare institutions and the evolving nature of healthcare settings, new quality assessment methods or tools should be incorporated into the clinical setting.

13.2   Quality Indicators: Types and Use in Healthcare Systems

Indicators have become the primary tool for the evaluation of healthcare systems and in turn foster their continuous improvement. Within the international context, databases such as the World Health Organization Global Health Observatory and the Economic Co-operation and Development Health Statistics play a major role in presenting global statics and indicators. Yet, to obtain precise and detailed information on a country level it is necessary to use suitable indicators able to assess a particular context. These indicators can vary between countries but may also overlap in certain instances due to their comprehensive nature. In particular the following examples of indicators may be considered:

1. *Indicators of the Agency for Healthcare Research and Quality* (AHRQ) [10], specifically the Inpatient Quality Indicators (IQI), Patient Safety Indicators (PSI), Preventive Quality Indicators (PQI) and the Pediatric Quality Indicators (PDI). These indicators are available on the website of the AHRQ, where the information and methodology to calculate these indicators is provided. One disadvantage of the AHRQ is that they lack comparison or benchmarking techniques between the indicators.
2. *MyNHS data-gathering platform* [11], which provides numerous performance indicators of health and social care services, and specifically compares hospital performance for 29 medical specialties. For each specialty they indicate the hospital performance and if their values are in the expected range compared to other hospitals. This tool is available to the public and is directed to inform citizens on hospital quality performance.
3. *Italian National Outcome Program* (Programma Nazionale Esiti, PNE) [12], a tool developed by the National Agency for Regional Healthcare Services (AGENAS) for a comparison between providers or Healthcare Agencies. The tool mainly focuses on outcome measurements, while also considering volume activity and other system measures.
4. *Sant'Anna School of Advanced Studies performance evaluation system of regional health systems* (Sistema di Valutazione delle Performance dei Sistemi Sanitari Regionali) [13], a voluntary evaluation tool used by over a dozen Italian

regions. The objective of this tool is to provide each region with a method for measuring, comparing and presenting the quality of the healthcare services offered by the region. The tool follows the Donabedian dimensions of care: structure, process and outcome [14].

The above-mentioned examples show how evaluation tools play an important role in assessing the quality of healthcare services. For each of these examples, there was a great effort to develop solid and specific indicators, but continuous collaborative efforts will be necessary also in the future to develop other pertinent indicators of outcome that can be used for benchmarking and continuous improvement.

Quality assessment is also advancing within the surgical field, with studies specifically investigating the relationship between outcome indicators and volume when assessing surgical safety. Some suggest that it may be best to monitor through risk-adjusted postoperative outcomes and investigate underperforming facilities [15], others that "the inverse association between high volume of procedure and risk of operative death is not specific to the volume of the procedure being studied" [16]. Indeed, this reasoning has led the PNE, which has numerous indicators related to oncological surgery, to develop outcome indicators together with volume indicators. Another very important methodology is the ACS National Surgical Quality Improvement Program ACS-NSQIP [17] that is a US validated, risk-adjusted, outcomes-based program to measure and improve the quality of surgical care. A study comparing the ACS-NSQIP [18] to the AHRQ-PSI, a tool widely recognized by surgeons, not only showed that the ACS methodology identified a larger number of adverse events but also shed light on the need for the use of more precise indicators.

13.3   New Technologies and Service Improvement

The evolution of the digital world in healthcare has deeply impacted accessibility to patient information and the analysis of medical data. This can be seen by the wide adoption of electronic health records (EHR) and electronic medical records (EMR) used by most hospitals in the USA (Fig. 13.1) [19], and across Europe [20, 21], with the European Union planning to expand EHR use even further under the European Commission recommendation 2019/243 [22]. Many other countries are also attempting to adopt EHR systems and evaluate the possibility of its diffusion based on factors such as costs and health information technology infrastructure [23, 24].

Other emerging technologies also include Clinical Decision Support Systems (CDSS) and machine learning and advanced analytics. CDSS is a software system that supports the decision-making of a clinician or healthcare professional, with its wide applicability impacting the delivery of primary and inpatient care and surgeries [25]. Machine learning and advanced analytics have allowed for real-time analysis and construct of predictions, which is more expedient compared to the more labor-intensive classical statistical tools used in the past. These technologies have been applied to the clinical setting and have allowed for more accurate EHR data

Fig. 13.1 Percentage of U.S. non-federal acute care hospitals (by type) that possess certified electronic health record technology (2017). (Source: https://dashboard.healthit.gov/quickstats/pages/certified-electronic-health-record-technology-in-hospitals.php)

assessments and predictions compared to the use of classical indicators and model-ing approaches [26].

Moreover, following the new digital era, organizations began providing services by using information and technology as tools to support healthcare transformation and improve health outcomes, as in the case of the Healthcare Information and Management Systems Society (HIMSS) [27]. HIMMS supports progress through technology adoption in healthcare and by following maturity models as tool to assess and enhance effectiveness. They propose models such as Electronic Medical Record Adoption Model (EMRAM) used by thousands of hospitals to incorporate electronic medical record, the Continuity of Care Maturity Model (CCMM) used to assess organizational progress capabilities, and the Adoption Model for Analytics Maturity (AMAM) used to measure and advance analytical capabilities.

All these facts help to understand how the digital world is something to face also in the healthcare context.

13.4   Classical Approach

Quality indicators mainly serve a statistical purpose, developed and used by hospi-tals and healthcare system administrators, researchers and policymakers who at times neglect the usefulness of these tools [28]. Differently, physicians and other healthcare professionals seem to prefer audit methodology as an approach to quality improvement as it often allows for a more in-depth analysis for fewer cases, a level of specificity deemed unnecessary for decision makers. These two approaches are often conducted in parallel, each suggesting different approaches for improvement, as shown in Figs. 13.2 and 13.3. Overcoming these differences is the first step towards a comprehensive implementation of clinical governance [29].

Fig. 13.2 Cycle of risk management. This cycle explains what is done on each event or near miss identified in a hospital. (Source: https://www.healthit.gov/topic/clinical-quality-and-safety)

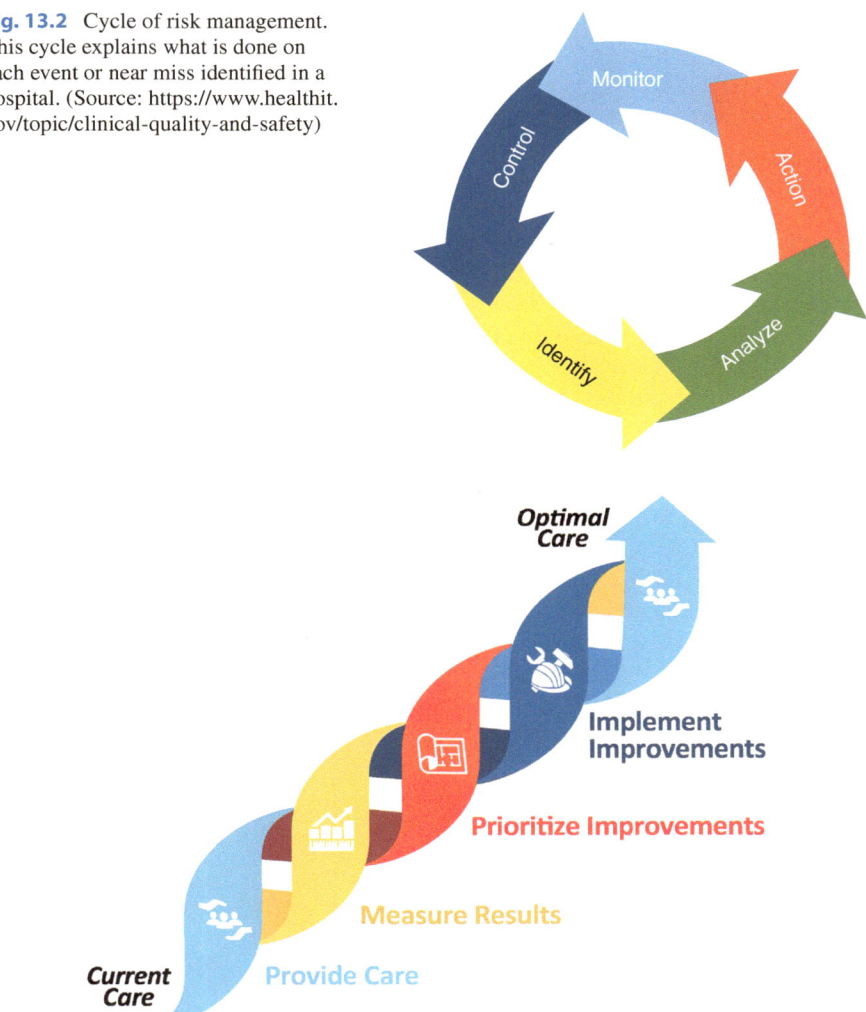

Fig. 13.3 Spiral of improvement through measures. The spiral in the image has, as an object, aggregated data around an area of care. (Source: https://www.healthit.gov/topic/clinical-quality-and-safety)

One way to merge these two process is by following the Institute of Health Care Improvement (IHI) Trigger Tool for Measuring Adverse Events [30]. The tool uses triggers (e.g., readmissions, infections, complications, return to surgery), normally part of quality indicators, which may be used at the decision level and may be applied to conduct auditing. However, this method seems no longer up to date as it does not involve new technological opportunities.

13.5   Combining Quality Indicators and Risk Management: Implementation

The main hypothetical approach to combine quality indicators and risk management methods is through technology. In other words, building a system that can constantly monitor quality indicators and drill down into case data (the numerator of indicators) in order to augment the potential of assessing and uncovering gaps through risk management methods. By using this approach not only is it possible to precisely determine the necessary improvement activities on a case-to-case basis, but also obtain a comprehensive view of the indicators measured allowing for a more effective prioritization of activities. A diagram of this approach is presented in Fig. 13.4.

In 2013, the Humanitas Clinical and Research Center implemented this system by integrating the following components:

- *Clinical Performance Information System* (CPIS): a web-based system able to manage and present all the indicators to every internal hospital user. The CPIS was introduced in July 2013 and the number of users has continued to increase, jumping from 600 to more than 2000 users in 2019. In 2014, 18% of total users accessed the system while 61% of users accessed it in 2019. The CPIS incorporates tables and graphs presenting the user with overall trends as well as the possibility to drill down into the case data. This allows for both the inclusion of indicator figures and the results form audits. The CPIS was developed to bridge such gaps.

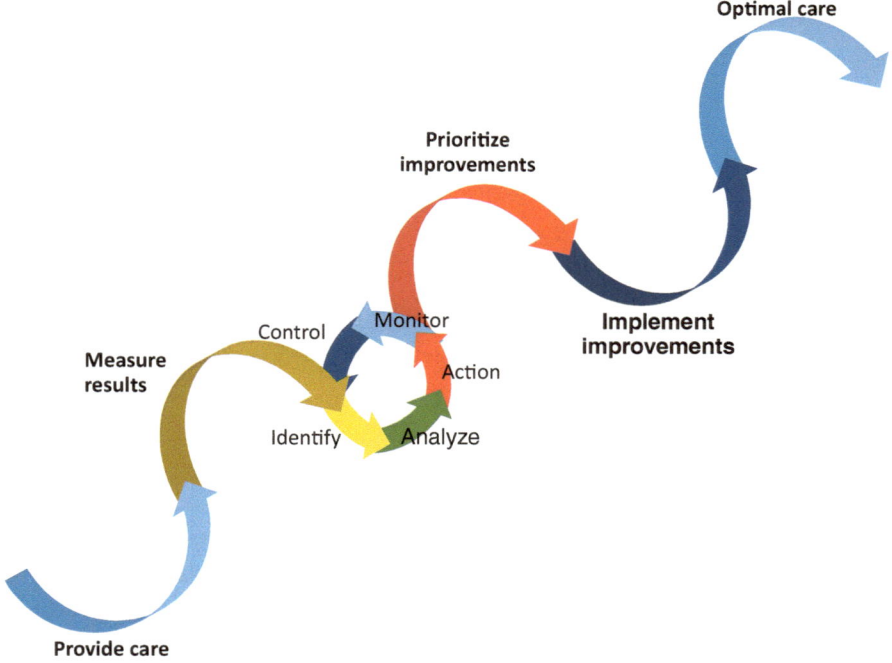

Fig. 13.4 Integration of risk management and measurement processes

- *Mortality Committee*: made up of approximately ten experts (active or retired chiefs of departments from all major hospital departments: cardiology, general surgery, general medicine, radiology, cardiac surgery, neurology, legal medicine, anesthesiology). Since 2013, these experts have met on a monthly basis to review, together with the patient's physician, all mortality cases from the previous month. The committee's objective is to assess the cause of death, determine if there were any issues related to the patient's safety and if there is any opportunity for improvement.
- *Malpractice Litigation Evaluation Committee*: was founded in 2009 while a major insurance company was still involved in the assessment and management of cases. In 2011 the committee reorganized, structurally similar to the mortality committee, with the aim of addressing the line of legal defense, but, more importantly, detecting the need for potential upgrades in quality of care.
- *Nurses' Improvement Committee*: started in December 2016 with the goal of assessing events or near misses involving nurses, and find the underlying causes of incidents and determine a strategy to avoid their reoccurrence.

The joint collaboration and work of all these activities allows for the development of solutions and new monitoring strategies. Often, the committee proposes process updates, the introduction of a new technology or the integration of specific indicators to enhance the monitoring of particular processes or outcomes. The introduction of new indicators can enable the committees to examine new types of cases creating a virtuous loop.

13.6   Combining Quality Indicators and Risk Management: Five Years' Experience

In-hospital elective surgery data from the Humanitas Clinical and Research Center was analyzed from January 2015 to June 2019. Because of the committees' focus on hospital patient mortality assessment, a decrease of in-hospital mortality was expected.

The data portrayed in Table 13.1 shows a decrease in elective surgery mortality. By using the APR-DRG (All Patient Refined-Diagnosis Related Groups, by 3M) weight, a classification system based on patients' reason for admission, it was

Table 13.1 Mortality, admissions, case-mix in surgical departments (2015–June 2019)

	Elective surgery			Emergency surgery	
Period	Number of admissions	In-hospital mortality (%)	APR-DRG	Number of admissions	In-hospital mortality (%)
2015	25,099	0.17	1.196538	1984	4.39
2016	26,686	0.17	1.218685	2039	4.32
2017	28,173	0.11	1.247753	2109	4.08
2018	29,450	0.08	1.246847	2116	4.40
Jan–June 2019	16,105	0.04	1.241795	1137	4.13

APR-DRG All Patient Refined-Diagnosis Related Groups

Table 13.2 Concentration of activities (Shannon index), case-mix (n. of cases, mean age), and related outcomes (2011–2015 and 2016–June 2019)

Period	Shannon index	Cases	Mean age	Length of stay	Mortality (%)	Re-operations (%)
2011–2015	5.879	14,022	57.24	8.50	3.72	3.40
2016–June 2019	5.522	9754	57.49	7.89	2.74	2.16

possible to further evaluate the severity of illness and risk of mortality measures. The results showed an increased weight, meaning that there is not any adverse selection of patients. Interestingly, the growing number of operations and decreasing mortality percentage suggest that the increase in number of elective surgeries does not necessarily prevent improvement in quality of care. This was not the case for emergency surgery mortality that remained stable throughout the studied period.

Importantly, these figures show the value of delivering indicator measurements to physicians and other health professionals, allowing the incorporation of their perspective and the possibility for them to apply surgical safety assessments and indications, avoiding the adverse selection of the case-mix.

To further elaborate on these results, a larger comparison was conducted starting from 2011 to June 2019 (Table 13.2), by including measure of distribution of intervention between different departments (calculated with the Shannon index [31]). The data was grouped from 2011 to 2015 and from 2016 to June 2019; as from 2015 a concentration of particular activities on specific departments was conducted to match patients' needs to the expertise of surgeons.

Looking at data from Table 13.2, we see how the effort to concentrate activities (Shannon index from 5879 to 5522) together with shifts in the approach to quality and risk management has led to reduced mortality and reoperations and shorter hospital length of stay during the 8-year period analyzed.

By conducting organizational changes and combining quality and risk management, the hospital was able to improve monitoring and to drive the actors involved in the development of hospital quality and safety to implement best solution for care.

In summary, combining the culture of numbers, by adopting suitable technology, together with the culture of safety, through risk management methodology, allows for healthcare delivery improvements. We aim to further use this method for two other phenomena: reoperations during the same admission and a sample of clinical pathways that needs renovation.

13.7 Further Remarks

In order to reach this state of continuous improvement, there are certain conditions that need to be met. Firstly, the hospital or healthcare system needs a strong managerial involvement, without which the decision-making process would be hindered through self-defined risk processes and ineffective change. Secondly, the hospital or healthcare systems should adopt relevant competencies for both risk management and use of quality indicators. These include skills in managing, analyzing and delivering data to involved stakeholders, as well as skills in risk management, collaboration with physicians and nurses, and delivering clinical governance. Thirdly, the hospital or healthcare system needs an advanced technological framework that enables and facilitates the collection and access of clinical data. This is important, as often EMR products may be difficult to use and acquire data from, inhibiting the continuous improvement process.

An important future outlook to consider is the acceptance of technological advancement within the evolving culture of care. The increasing number of tools able to conduct real-time assessments and recommendations allow for more effective advancements, yet their impact might be limited as healthcare professionals are not prone to use them. One solution would be to foster the collaboration of technicians and informaticians with healthcare professionals in the development of such tools.

13.8 Conclusions

Through this chapter we observed two approaches to determine the best outcomes of healthcare provision. On the one hand, we showed that examining the volume-outcome relationship aims to find an easy way to reach the best outcome, and so, if the relationship exists, it is simpler to look at volume to reach a better outcome. On the other hand, we explained how the use of both a quantitative and empirical approach could also determine better outcomes, specifically by combining quality indicators and risk management methods through technology.

It is important to acknowledge these different approaches and consider the possibility of connecting their methodologies, as they are not exclusive but rather can complement one another. To develop new tools and solutions, it is crucial to envisage the use of new technologies with the aim of supporting healthcare professionals in putting in place immediate control measures and advancements.

References

1. Som CV. Clinical governance: a fresh look at its definition. Clin Gov. 2004;9(2):87–90. https://doi.org/10.1108/14777270410536358.
2. Gottwald M, Lansdown GE. Clinical governance: improving the quality of healthcare for patients and service users. 1st ed. Maidenhead: McGraw-Hill Education; 2014.
3. Dyer C. Bristol inquiry: Bristol inquiry condemns hospital's "club culture". BMJ. 2001;323(7306):181.
4. Kohn LT, Corrigan JM, Donaldson MS, editors; Committee on Quality of Health Care in America—Institute of Medicine. To err is human. Building a safer health system. Washington, DC: National Academies Press; 2000. https://www.ncbi.nlm.nih.gov/books/NBK225182/pdf/Bookshelf_NBK225182.pdf.
5. Institute for Healthcare Improvement (IHI). History. http://www.ihi.org/about/Pages/History.aspx.

6. Joint Commission International (JCI). Who we are. https://www.jointcommissioninterna-tional.org/about-jci/who-we-are.
7. Kaya GK. The relationship between risk management and patient safety incidents in acute hospitals in NHS England. In: Calisir F, Cevikcan E, Camgoz Akdag H, editors. Industrial engineering in the big data era. Cham: Springer; 2019.
8. NIHR Global Health Research Unit on Global Surgery. Quality and outcomes in global cancer surgery: protocol for a multicentre, international, prospective cohort study (GlobalSurg 3). BMJ Open. 2019;9(5):e026646. https://doi.org/10.1136/bmjopen-2018-026646.
9. Spark JI, Rowe S. Clinical governance: its effect on surgery and the surgeon. ANZ J Surg. 2004;74(3):167–70.
10. Agency for Healthcare Research and Quality. Quality indicators. https://www.qualityindica-tors.ahrq.gov.
11. National Health Service. MyNHS website. Data on speciality treatments. https://www.nhs.uk/mynhs/specialties.html.
12. Agenzia Nazionale dei Servizi Sanitari Regionale (AGENAS). Programma Nazionale Esiti (PNE). https://pne.agenas.it.
13. Scuola Superiore Sant'Anna di Pisa. Sistema di Valutazione delle Performance dei Sistemi Sanitari Regionali. http://performance.sssup.it/netval/start.php.
14. Donabedian A. Evaluating the quality of medical care. Milbank Mem Fund Q. 1966;44(3 Pt 2):166–206. Reprinted in: Milbank Q. 2005;83(4):691–729.
15. Eggli Y, Halfon P, Meylan D, Taffé P. Surgical safety and hospital volume across a wide range of interventions. Med Care. 2010;48(11):962–71.
16. Urbach DR, Baxter NN. Does it matter what a hospital is "high volume" for? Specificity of hospital volume-outcome associations for surgical procedures: analysis of administrative data. Qual Saf Health Care. 2004;13:379–83.
17. American College of Surgeon. ACS National Surgical Quality Improvement Program (ACS NSQIP). https://www.facs.org/quality-programs/acs-nsqip.
18. Cima RR, Lackore KA, Nehring SA, et al. How best to measure surgical quality? Comparison of the Agency for Healthcare Research and Quality Patient Safety Indicators (AHRQ-PSI) and the American College of Surgeons National Surgical Quality Improvement Program (ACS-NSQIP) postoperative adverse events at a single institution. Surgery. 2011;150(5):943–9.
19. The Office of the National Coordinator for Health Information Technology. Health IT Dashboard. Quick Stats. https://dashboard.healthit.gov/quickstats/quickstats.php.
20. From innovation to implementation: eHealth in the WHO European Region. World Health Organization; 2016. http://www.euro.who.int/__data/assets/pdf_file/0012/302331/From-Innovation-to-Implementation-eHealth-Report-EU.pdf?ua=1.
21. Adoption and use of electronic medical records and e-prescribing. In: OECD/European Union. Health at a glance: Europe 2018. Paris: OECD Publishing; 2019. p. 192–3. https://doi.org/10.1787/health_glance_eur-2018-56-en.
22. Commission Recommendation on a European Electronic Health Record exchange format (C(2019)800) of 6 February 2019. https://ec.europa.eu/newsroom/dae/document.cfm?doc_id=57253 (annex: https://ec.europa.eu/newsroom/dae/document.cfm?doc_id=57254).
23. Lee YT, Park YT, Park JS, Yi BK. Association between electronic medical record system adoption and healthcare information technology infrastructure. Healthc Inform Res. 2018;24(4):327–34.
24. Heimly V, Grimsmo A, Faxvaag A. Diffusion of electronic health records and electronic communication in Norway. Appl Clin Inform. 2011;2(3):355–64.
25. Berlin A, Sorani M, Sim I. A taxonomic description of computer-based clinical decision support systems. J Biomed Inform. 2006;39(6):656–67.
26. Rajkomar A, Oren E, Chen K, et al. Scalable and accurate deep learning with electronic health records. NPJ Digit Med. 2018;1:18. https://doi.org/10.1038/s41746-018-0029-1.
27. Healthcare Information and Management Systems Society, Inc. (HIMSS). Who we are. https://www.himss.org/who-we-are.

28. Jha A, Epstein A. Hospital governance and the quality of care. Health Aff (Millwood). 2010;29(1):182–7.
29. Degeling PJ, Maxwell S, Iedema R, Hunter DJ. Making clinical governance work. BMJ. 2004;329(7467):679–81.
30. Griffin FA, Resar RK. IHI Global Trigger Tool for measuring adverse events. 2nd ed. Cambridge, MA: Institute for Healthcare Improvement; 2009.
31. Shannon CE, Weaver W. The mathematical theory of communication. Urbana, IL: The University of Illinois Press; 1949.

Centralization in Surgery in European Countries

14

René Vonlanthen, Samuel Käser, and Pierre-Alain Clavien

14.1 Introduction

European countries are challenged by the growing costs of their health care systems. The issue is complex due to numerous factors and perspectives involved in a market which includes various players and conflicting interests. These factors are further influenced by country-specific circumstances, like geopolitical conditions, available resources and social values. Patient-perceived values, integrated today in concepts of value-based medicine [1, 2], are rarely at the center of the debate, although quality of care with endpoints relevant to patients and to the whole society are gaining increasing attention.

High quality of health care at reasonable cost is the target of all accountable health care systems, but the definition of quality remains vague and therefore subjected to versatile interpretation. An important question is how to provide high quality complex procedural care with policies ranging from unregulated free markets to centralization (regionalization) in a single national center. Centralization is a process of concentration of resources, which includes infrastructure, staff, material, knowledge, and research. This process is believed to lead to improved quality of care and ultimately to enhanced financial efficiency. How centralization should be implemented remains a controversy and in many countries the focus lays on centralization of complex surgical procedures.

Today, many elements have been established in the surgical field that are associated with incremental improvements in the quality of surgical care [3]. One repeated observation is that high-volume institutions are associated with improved outcome through appropriate and better indications, surgical procedures, and postoperative management [4, 5]. Additional key factors for better outcome are surgeon volume, specialization and the so-called "rescue phenomenon", meaning the ability to

R. Vonlanthen · S. Käser · P.-A. Clavien (✉)

Department of Surgery and Transplantation, University Hospital Zurich, Zurich, Switzerland
e-mail: rene.vonlanthen@usz.ch; samuel.kaeser@usz.ch; clavien@access.uzh.ch

© Springer Nature Switzerland AG 2021
M. Montorsi (ed.), *Volume-Outcome Relationship in Oncological Surgery*,
Updates in Surgery, https://doi.org/10.1007/978-3-030-51806-6_14

prevent minor postoperative events developing into severe complications and death [6]. Recently it has been demonstrated that operating on complex and not only on "standard cases" (benchmark cases) is key for a qualitatively successful surgical program [7].

14.2 Centralization Policies in Europe: General Overview

The European Observatory on Health Systems and Policies has demonstrated the diversity and different rates of progress in developing a concept of reference centers and networks in Europe. In some countries, centralization is mainly driven by limitation of the number of medical institutions, in others by the desire to improve clinical expertise and research on the treatment of specific (mainly rare) diseases. Some countries have developed well-established systems for monitoring activities and outcomes in specific fields (e.g., cancer), and others have just historically established leading centers of excellence to which patients are referred, without any clear criteria or quality control mechanisms. In the field of critical care (transplants, burns), networks are often especially built around a central coordination center.

Two main concepts have emerged: (1) the concentration of expertise and care on the one hand, and (2) the transfer of this expertise between and within networks on the other. To a certain extent these concepts are in competition with each other. At the level of the European Union the development of European reference networks (ERNs) is planned to improve access to and provision of high-quality health care to all patients. These networks could act as focal points for medical training and research, information dissemination and evaluation, especially for rare diseases. The aim is to facilitate also access to safe and high-quality cross-border health care. But we are still not so far.

14.3 Centralization Policies in Europe with Focus on Gastrointestinal Surgery

Nearly 50 years after the landmark publication by Luft et al. [8] on regionalization of surgical care, only little progress can be observed in Europe [7]. Centralization policies in surgery are implemented mainly by the definition of minimal volume numbers in terms of activity per center for selective procedures in 13 of 20 (65%) investigated European countries, and only 5% (1/20) have proposed a minimal case load per surgeon (Table 14.1). Four countries, the Czech Republic, Greece, Poland and Romania have currently no policy regarding centralization in gastrointestinal surgery.

Procedures or diseases to be centralized are defined differently by health care policy makers, typically national and regional governments. For example, Austria, Denmark, and Switzerland based their choices for centralization on rarity of the disease, complexity with high postoperative morbidity, structural requirements and

Table 14.1 Requirement for minimal numbers (resections/year) per center [7]

Country	Esophagus	Pancreas	Liver	Rectum	Surgeon volume	Legally enforced
Austria	10	10	10 (20 [a])	10 (15 [a])	ND	Yes
Belgium	ND	ND	ND	ND	ND	
Czech Republic	ND	ND	ND	ND	ND	
Denmark [b]	80–100	>100	>200	>120	ND	
England (UK) [b]	60	80	150	ND	1	
Finland	ND	ND	ND	ND	ND	
France [c]	30	30	30	30	ND	Yes
Germany	10	10	ND	ND	ND	Yes
Greece	15	20	30	ND	ND	
Hungary	10	20	30	20	ND	
Ireland [b]	ND	ND	ND	ND	ND	
Italy	20	50–100	20	50	ND	
Norway [b]	10	10	20	20	ND	
Poland	ND	ND	ND	ND	ND	
Portugal	20	20	20	20	ND	
Romania	ND	ND	ND	ND	ND	
Spain	6	11	11	15	ND	Yes
Sweden [b]	ND	ND	ND	ND	ND	
Switzerland	10	10	10	10	ND	Yes
The Netherlands	20	20	20	20	ND	Yes

ND not defined

[a]Year 2018

[b]Not based on minimal numbers, but defined catchment areas/health care regions. Denmark, England and Norway have additionally secured minimal numbers

[c]In France minimal number of 30 procedures in total for cancer irrespective of the location

costs, and on scientific evidence for a volume-outcome relationship. In other countries, complexity, management with multiple disciplines and technical challenges of the procedures followed by financial burden are the most common factors, recognizing a need for centralization for procedures on the esophagus, pancreas, liver, and rectum. Centralization policies may either relate to technical procedures on an organ, or be restricted to specific cancers (e.g., pancreatic cancer) or conditions, such as morbid obesity. So, centralization in surgery has been undertaken across European countries based on different concepts.

Furthermore, there is an obvious discrepancy between regulations for centralization and implementation. For instance, volume thresholds in Austria and Germany are not respected despite requirements clearly set out by the law. While centralization is well implemented in the field of transplantation, burns, pediatric and neurosurgery, the reality is very different for gastrointestinal procedures. A recent study on the centralization of pancreatic surgery in Europe shows that European countries have failed to establish centralization to high-volume centers for numerous reasons and the review enforces the worldwide plea for centralization to lower postoperative mortality after pancreatic surgery [9]. The Netherlands, the UK and Denmark are good examples of a strong centralization and good performance.

14.4 Examples of Centralization Policies in European Countries

14.4.1 Denmark

Denmark counts five health care regions today. Each region operates a public hospital and has a university hospital. This is the result of a radical restructuring that was accompanied by important financial investments.

The Danish health authority regulates and coordinates highly specialized services including complex abdominal operations. According to this regulation, (highly) specialized abdominal operations are performed in 1–4 locations across the country, whereas there exists a cooperation between regions. Of note, despite the small population size, the minimum number of cases is the highest in Europe (Table 14.1; e.g., esophagus 80–100/year; pancreas >100/year). A recent national study demonstrated a slight improvement in survival and relative mortality in pancreatic cancer, which may well reflect the national cancer centralization strategy [10].

14.4.2 England and Scotland

Health policies in England (80% of the population), Scotland, Wales and Northern Ireland are different. The main policy in England has been towards more decentralization, reinforcement of the internal market, and more localized decision-making. Scotland and Wales have moved in the other direction, dissolving the internal market and keeping more power centralized.

14.4.2.1 England

Major hospitals bid to the NHS (National Health System) England for funds to provide services. England also uses payment systems intended to create incentives for quality and efficiency, that is, a "Payment by Results" and "Pay for Performance" system linking a small proportion of provider income to certain goals. Since 2001 and according to a guide on the development of cancer networks, cancer teams should have a catchment area of two to four million inhabitants [11]. Today (highly) specialized services are provided by only a few hospitals. Based on different criteria, specialized services are commissioned directly by the NHS as it is for liver, pancreas, esophagus, and lower rectum resections, and for bariatric surgery or, when the criteria not met, by Clinical Commission Groups. A key body is the National Institute for Health and Care Excellence (NICE), which advises on the cost-effectiveness of interventions. NICE plays an important role for publication of pathways, guidance, standards, and indicators and, as of April 2013, NICE took over the role of the AGNSS (Advisory Group for National Specialized Services) in appraising highly specialized technologies. "NHS England current national specifications" recommend minimal case volumes for multidisciplinary teams (without legal enforcement) (Table 14.1). Specialized cancer networks have developed based on a hub-and-spoke model and through centralization, many surgeons lost their "cancer work" and are forced to operate in their nearby associated centers and continuing to provide general surgery services at their local hospitals [12, 13]. Centralization of esophagogastric cancer resulted in England in a reduction of the 30-day mortality rate from 7.4 to 2.5% [14]. and in pancreatic surgery 30-day mortality in England decreased from 6.2 to 5.7% between 1999 and 2005, while hospitals performing pancreatic resections decreased from 101 to 73 and annual cases increased from 1473 to 1905. NHS England has designed policies to monitor contracted hospital trusts to verify adherence to the volume indicators.

14.4.2.2 Scotland

Boards and community health partnerships manage their own funds in Scotland and use a capitation-based allocation system. Scottish continuous peer review audits and studies analyzing patients managed in high-volume centers and by specialists showed significantly improved outcome [15]. These data triggered the establishment of the Managed Clinical Network patterns coordinated by an Executive Board. The duty of this network is to organize the specialized units within a network [13]. The network defines also national guidelines, ensures the appointment of clinical nurse practitioners in each unit, and undertakes regular audits of practice.

14.4.3 Finland

Finland is a sparsely populated country with a well-established strong decentralization of health care services. The situation is planned to be reversed, as the country has become increasingly concerned about geographical inequalities in access to health care. In the north distance to the nearest high-volume center is over 500 km. Irrespective of this fact centralization of pancreatic surgery has proceeded gradually in Finland since the 1990s. In a recent study from national registers it has been shown that both short- and long-term survival was significantly better for patients operated in high volume centers [16]. Finland may become in the future an example of centralization of surgical care in a big but sparsely populated country.

14.4.4 France

French hospital facilities need to perform a minimum annual number of 30 procedures for breast, digestive, urologic and thoracic cancers and of 20 procedures for gynecologic and ear-nose-throat (ENT) cancers. These criteria have been implemented to ensure that quality of cancer care is guaranteed and, amongst others, that each patient is discussed at a multidisciplinary team meeting. This volume regulation has allowed a reduction in the number of facilities with (very) low annual caseloads of cancer surgery. However, a recent study in pancreatic surgery underlines that centralization has not actually occurred and the majority of patients are operated on in low-volume centers [17]. A radical centralization of pancreatic resections is currently hardly feasible due to high-volume units being limited in number and unevenly distributed throughout France. The same applies to liver surgery [18].

14.4.5 Germany

The German Federal Joint Committee established minimum caseload requirements for several procedures in 2004 [19]. Currently, this regulation covers seven procedures, two of which in abdominal surgery. A minimal caseload of ten cases per year is required for complex esophageal and pancreatic operations [20], knowing that still 25% of German hospitals only perform one or two pancreatic resections per year.

Surprisingly, German single-center studies suggest acceptable or even excellent outcome after surgery. Nationwide this is not the case as has been shown and confirmed in different studies [21, 22]. Among 18,000 patients (data from 2009 to 2014) undergoing esophageal resection for carcinoma in Germany, the adjusted mortality rate was 5.8% (95% CI 5.1–6.6) on the very high-volume quintile vs. 10.5% (9.5–11.6%) in the very low quintile. Hospital volume had an independent effect on mortality, and the minimum volume to fall below the average mortality of 8.5% was calculated as 22 cases per year [23]. National observational studies demonstrated a lower risk of in-hospital death for hospitals adhering to the minimal caseload requirements of 10/year [23, 24]. It was calculated that in Germany centralizing pancreatic procedures could save around 300 lives per year [20]. Minimal volume numbers should be legally enforced on a national level but are ignored by many providers as this rarely has economic consequences [25]. This reflects a structural problem as the German hospital landscape is characterized by overcapacity and too many small, non-specialized hospitals [26]. According to a recent study three steps are imperative towards the introduction of centralization in Germany: a significant increase of the annual minimal caseload, consequent enforcement of these regulations and no granting of exceptions [9].

14.4.6 Ireland

In Ireland in 2006 eight cancer centers were defined whereas surgery for some cancer types is restricted to two (pancreas) or four (esophagus, gastric) specialized centers. There is no formal centralization for liver cancer surgery, although only three centers in Ireland have liver surgical programs.

14.4.7 Italy

In Italy, the outcome of pancreaticoduodenectomy in 2003 was significantly dependent on hospital volume. Hence, it was suggested that a policy of centralization may be appropriate [27]. Since 2009, Italian hospitals are evaluated by the National

Outcome Program, which also monitors volume indicators [28]. In parallel, the Italian Society of Surgery has attempted to define criteria identifying hospitals able to perform complex gastrointestinal procedures [29]. They have made specific proposals for esophageal [30], hepatic [31], pancreatic [29] and colorectal [32] surgery. The minimal numbers listed for Italy represent recommendations rather than mandatory figures (Table 14.1). A centralized model for complex surgeries in Italy is unlikely to be realized due to socioeconomic factors [33].

14.4.8 Norway

Norway's health system is under the control of four Regional Health Authorities (RHA) of diverse population density, geographical distances, variable inhabitant numbers, and absolute number of procedures performed. Recommendations and guidelines for cancer surgery were issued by the Norwegian Directory of Health in a report in 2015 [34], but there are no enforcements for specified minimal volume numbers (Table 14.1). The report foresees a multidisciplinary team approach for cancer care and recently a strong centralization was implemented for most cancer types. For example, liver and pancreas cancer surgery is restricted to five hospitals and esophageal cancer surgery to four hospitals. Each RHA is responsible for the implementation, governance and monitoring of cancer surgery and this is usually repeated in a 4-year review cycle.

In-hospital mortality for pancreatoduodenectomy in Norway (2012–2016) was at 2% and the 90-day mortality rate was low (4%) [35]. This good outcome may reflect the centralization of pancreatic surgery. Importantly, the resection rates per inhabitant number (i.e., population-based incidence of resections) are equal across all regions suggesting an equal service provided to the population [35].

14.4.9 Spain

Spain is decentralized and has 17 regional health authorities. As an example, the Catalan Health Service (CatSalut) has imposed centralization for digestive oncologic surgeries in 2005 [36], which was further reinforced in 2012 by a directive that assigned a very limited number of centers for complex cancer interventions based on minimal volume of cases and specialization criteria. Peritoneal carcinomatosis surgery, retroperitoneal or neuroendocrine tumor management are further examples of centralized care organization.

Positive effects of centralization were observed, with reduction of mortality rates in esophageal and pancreatic oncologic surgery [36]. Short- and long-term quality improvements by centralization and audits were also documented for rectal cancer surgery [37, 38]. Audits are performed in Catalonia by the Director of the Oncologic Plan every year and results are communicated to each audited center. If an intervention is performed in a hospital not holding a proper mandate, reimbursement is denied.

14.4.10 Sweden

Sweden has six Regional Cancer Centers (RCCs) since 2011. The role of this orga-nization is to contribute to more equitable, safe, and effective cancer care through regional and national collaboration. Specialized abdominal cancer surgery is there-fore concentrated to one unit of each of the six RCCs. Thus, depending on the size of the RCC, one hospital for abdominal cancer has a catchment area of one to three million inhabitants. However, no minimal numbers are defined for cancer surgery. On a national level ten tumor types and surgical procedures have been concentrated in two hospitals with a catchment area of five million inhabitants; for gastrointesti-nal cancer these are: locally advanced pancreatic cancer, advanced esophageal can-cer, perihilar bile duct cancer, anal cancer, and liver transplantation. Hyperthermic intraperitoneal chemotherapy (HIPEC) is still performed in four hospitals.

In a recent Swedish study long-term survival was improved at higher volume hospitals for some gastrointestinal cancers (colon, esophagus, pancreas, rectum), but not for others (stomach, liver, bile ducts, small bowel) [39]. In another study the best predictor of outcome was "teaching hospital" status. The hospital status likely serves as an indicator for hospitals with a more complex service and several disci-plines available to handle complications around the hour [40].

14.4.11 Switzerland

Switzerland's health care system is characterized by a strong decentralized policy. The 26 cantons have the authority and autonomy on health care delivery in their territory except for highly specialized medicine (HSM), which is regulated by the Swiss government (https://www.gdk-cds.ch). Five gastrointestinal operations belong to HSM including esophageal, pancreatic, liver, and rectal resections, as well as bariatric surgery. In 2012, the minimal volume numbers of ten procedures per year were required in each category. Several hospitals with borderline or with-out a mandate for HSM interventions appealed at the federal court and succeeded in delaying the implementation of the required minimal case volumes for some time.

A recent published population-based analysis demonstrates a higher postopera-tive mortality in low-volume hospitals for patients undergoing esophageal, gastric, pancreatic and rectal cancer resection in Switzerland [41].

14.4.12 The Netherlands

The Dutch example offers an interesting setting to evaluate the use of minimum volume standards and centralization effects over a 14-year period (2003–2017) [42]. In 1993, an influential report on the quality and distribution of cancer care was published, which triggered nationwide agreements on concentration of complex cancer care. Before introducing official thresholds by health policy makers, regional hospitals cooperated to simulate centralization on a regional level. However, it took

10 years (2003) until the first minimal volume indicators were enforced for operations on abdominal aortic aneurysm and on esophageal cancer. In 2009, some health insurers started contracting based on quality indicators (e.g., volume standards) and raised the "quality bar" to distinguish themselves from their competitors. Minimal volume criteria for pancreatic resections followed in 2010. This process of enforcement of minimal volume numbers was further accompanied by mainstream media activity that raised the awareness of the public for health performance indicators. Meanwhile, and partly in response to this development, medical associations published sets of comprehensive norms, including minimum volume standards. Along the same line, insurance providers generally comply with the same minimum volume standards as recommended by the professionals' associations. In 2014 and 2015, the nationwide mortality rate after pancreatic resections was 3.6% compared to 9.8% in 2004. Apart from a decrease in general mortality a major benefit for elderly patients ($\geq$75 years) was demonstrated. The excellent outcome of this initiative has led to a further debate on increasing the threshold to 40 or even 60 annual pancreatectomies.

14.5 Effect of Different Factors on Centralization

High hospital and surgeon volume are relevant factors that affect outcome positively. Based on these findings there has been a growing tendency to centralize complex surgical care in high-volume centers such as esophageal and pancreatic resections. Cut-offs for the definition of high-volume centers and minimal surgeon volume present a wide range indicating that other key factors than these have a positive impact on outcome, including specialization, care by multidisciplinary teams, coverage by specialists 24 h a day, specialized intensive care units, board-certified intensivists, and high nurse-to-patient ratios. The relation between volume and outcome may follow two scenarios: outcome parameters may follow a plateau after reaching a certain volume threshold or may be associated with poorer results, for example, when the infrastructure is at its limit. These has been extensively discussed in a recent paper [7].

Another mechanism for improved outcome at larger centers is the concept of "failure to rescue". Although low- and high-volume hospitals may have comparable complication rates, high-volume hospitals have a 2.5 × lower mortality rate. An explanation therefore might be that high-volume hospitals have more resources which grant the ability to rescue a patient from major complications [6].

14.6 Patient Perspective on Centralization

In a Swedish study the most relevant factor in the patient's perspective on centralization is quality of care (outcome) [43]. Additional factors such as well-functioning care pathways, individualized care plans, continuity of treatment with local providers, accessibility for contact and information, involvement in the care process, and limited waiting time are also important for patient satisfaction. One disadvantage of centralization is an increase in travel demands, therefore also perceived as limited access to high-quality care with greater distance from relatives. So, patients in England were willing to travel on average 75 min longer in order to reduce their risk of complications by 1%, and over 5 h longer to reduce risk of death by 1% [44]. In cancer services in England factors that matter to patients and health care professionals are: highly trained staff, likelihood and severity of complications, waiting time for cancer surgery, and access to staff members form various disciplines with specialized skills in cancer care [45]. The different stakeholder groups identified similar factors as being important but there was considerable heterogeneity in ordering the relevance of these factors.

According to studies from the USA patients' hospital selection by outcome data might be overestimated [46, 47]. In the case of centralization, travel patterns [48], socioeconomic status (e.g., household income) and race [49] have to be considered in multicultural countries such as the USA [50, 51]. These findings may also apply to European countries.

14.7   Surgeons' Perspective on Centralization

Dutch surgeons have gained experience of volume-based policies over the past two decades [52]. The majority supports that more volume leads to better outcome after surgery. They critically emphasize, however, that hospital volume is more a surrogate marker for the quality of the infrastructure and processes, rather than the performance of individual surgeons. Many surgeons complained about the arbitrary nature of the centralization process due to the under-representation of surgeons in the national committees that define the volume bar. Criticisms were also raised that volume bar levels were set without sufficient evidence. Furthermore, several committee members had obvious conflict of interest as they were employees of high-volume centers. Another complaint related to the "gate to surgery", i.e., indications, which became a little wider to reach the requested volume threshold. Most of interviewed surgeons also criticize the attitude of health insurers in misusing volume discussions to increase pressure on health care providers.

14.8   Centralization and Surgical Training

Moving toward centralization means also facing new challenges for proper training and the requirement for the development of harmonized models for the training of the next generation of medical specialists. The Union Européene des Médecins

Spécialistes (UEMS; www.uems.eu) contributed to the improvement for postgraduate training through the development of a European Curriculum in each medical specialty. Today more than 30 disciplines have European examinations. While they are still not to be considered formal qualifications, some countries recognize European examinations today as part of their national examination (e.g., Switzerland). However, accreditation of training programs with formalized and quality-controlled fellowship training as in the USA is still in early development. The need for designated and specialized post-residency training is evident in the USA with more than 70% of residents entering a formal training program in a surgical specialty after residency [53].

The tremendous and incessant advances in novel technology (e.g., robotics) requires continuing medical education and continuing professional development to secure optimal patient care. Here the importance of postgraduate education and the increasing need for training and accreditation for new technical skills cannot be overemphasized.

In parallel, working hour restrictions, as implemented in many countries, make adequate and timely surgical and subspecialty training increasingly difficult [53]. Further we notice in most European countries that the total number of hospitals is decreasing. These developments imply that postgraduate training must be guided and monitored on a national level. Highly specialized procedures should be performed exclusively in a restricted number of centers and by surgeons with extra—and possibly accredited—training in a specific area of surgery. But complex procedures should not be excluded from "general" surgical training. An adequate balance of general and specialized surgeons must be well planned in a health care system to maintain accessibility to high-quality health care in all geographic areas in a country. Networking between highly specialized institutions and other hospitals seems to be a factor to optimize accessibility of care to patients.

14.9   Recommendations for Centralization in Surgery in Europe

In 2018, Members of the European Surgical Association (ESA) presented 12 recommendations (Table 14.2) for centralization in surgery at their annual meeting. The proposal based on a Delphi process came after an intensive review of the available data regarding volume-outcome, failure to rescue, and benchmark studies. The recommendations are simple statements applicable to various health care systems in Europe and may serve as a basis for discussions in various areas to improve health care delivery (Table 14.2) [7].

Table 14.2 Recommendations for centralization [7]

Definition	1.	**Definition of diseases or interventions to centralize** Based on disease (e.g. pancreatic cancer) or on organ systems (e.g. complex HPB diseases) rather than a procedure (e.g. esophagus, pancreas resection)
Planning	2.	**Planning of catchment areas (e.g. one to five million inhabitants)** rather than planning on minimal numbers
	3.	**Planning of at least two centers per country** to secure choice and competition
Resources	4.	**Secure appropriate resources** Evaluation of availability of infrastructure and personnel, interdisciplinary teams of well-trained specialists (24 h a day, every day)
Network	5.	**Develop network activities for proper referral and follow-up**
Implementation	6.	**Specifications of centralization are legally enforced** Adherence to specifications is mandatory on a local and regional level and for the private and non-private sector
Information-PR	7.	**Whole process is accompanied by mainstream media activities**
Quality control	8.	**Centers have an externally audited database**
	9.	**Quality control is accompanied by international benchmark comparative studies**
	10.	**Equal accessibility to health care is monitored**
Research	11.	**Centers conduct prospective clinical studies and should be encouraged to perform basic research, or at least collaborate with basic scientists**
Education	12.	**Centralized national planning of surgical education** Centers secure specialized training and allow also rotation of "general surgeons"

HPB hepatopancreatobiliary, *PR* public relations

14.10 Conclusion

In conclusion, centralization and volume-outcome data are inherently associated with some limitations. Studies in this field are mostly observational, retrospective, and are based on administrative data collected for other purposes. Centralization policies are more or less implemented in many European countries but are not readily found in the literature, which makes comprehensive overviews difficult [7, 35]. The process of centralization is obviously of great importance to offer better care to patients suffering from complex diseases requiring special expertise and costly technology. Patient and health care professionals have similar perspectives in this regard but there is a certain heterogeneity in ordering the relevance of these factors. The 12 recommendations of the ESA members may serve as a basis for discussion in various areas to improve health care delivery.

References

1. Stapleton SM, Chang DC, Rattner DW, Ferris TG. Along for the ride? Surgeon participation in accountable care organizations. Ann Surg. 2018;267(3):408–10.

2. Resnick MJ, Graves AJ, Buntin MB, et al. Surgeon participation in early accountable care organizations. Ann Surg. 2018;267(3):401–7.
3. Clavien PA. Targeting quality in surgery. Ann Surg. 2013;258(5):659–68.
4. Mesman R, Westert GP, Berden BJ, Faber MJ. Why do high-volume hospitals achieve better outcomes? A systematic review about intermediate factors in volume-outcome relationships. Health Policy. 2015;119(8):1055–67.
5. Nguyen YL, Wallace DJ, Yordanov Y, et al. The volume-outcome relationship in critical care: a systematic review and meta-analysis. Chest. 2015;148(1):79–92.
6. Ghaferi AA, Birkmeyer JD, Dimick JB. Complications, failure to rescue, and mortality with major inpatient surgery in Medicare patients. Ann Surg. 2009;250(6):1029–34.
7. Vonlanthen R, Lodge P, Barkun JS, et al. Toward a consensus on centralization in surgery. Ann Surg. 2018;268(5):712–24.
8. Luft HS, Bunker JP, Enthoven AC. Should operations be regionalized? The empirical relation between surgical volume and mortality. N Engl J Med. 1979;301(25):1364–9.
9. Polonski A, Izbicki JR, Uzunoglu FG. Centralization of pancreatic surgery in Europe. J Gastrointest Surg. 2019;23(10):2081–92.
10. Cronin-Fenton DP, Erichsen R, Mortensen FV, et al. Pancreatic cancer survival in central and northern Denmark from 1998 through 2009: a population-based cohort study. Clin Epidemiol. 2011;3(Suppl 1):19–25.
11. Urbach DR. Pledging to eliminate low-volume surgery. N Engl J Med. 2015;373(15):1388–90.
12. Siriwardena AK. Centralisation of upper gastrointestinal cancer surgery. Ann R Coll Surg Engl. 2007;89(4):335–6.
13. Mole DJ, Parks RW. Centralization of surgery for pancreatic cancer. In: Büchler MW, Shrikhande SV, editors. Surgery of pancreatic cancer: current issues. New Delhi: Elsevier; 2012.
14. Varagunam M, Hardwick R, Riley S, et al. Changes in volume, clinical practice and outcome after reorganisation of oesophago-gastric cancer care in England: a longitudinal observational study. Eur J Surg Oncol. 2018;44(4):524–31.
15. Young J, Thompson A, Tait I, et al. Centralization of services and reduction of adverse events in pancreatic cancer surgery. World J Surg. 2013;37(9):2229–33.
16. Ahola R, Siiki A, Vasama K, et al. Effect of centralization on long-term survival after resection of pancreatic ductal adenocarcinoma. Br J Surg. 2017;104(11):1532–8.
17. Farges O, Bendersky N, Truant S, et al. The theory and practice of pancreatic surgery in France. Ann Surg. 2017;266(5):797–804.
18. Farges O, Goutte N, Dokmak S, et al. How surgical technology translates into practice: the model of laparoscopic liver resections performed in France. Ann Surg. 2014;260(5):916–21; discussion 921–2.
19. Peschke D, Nimptsch U, Mansky T. Achieving minimum caseload requirements—an analysis of hospital discharge data from 2005–2011. Dtsch Arztebl Int. 2014;111(33–34):556–63.
20. Baltin CT, Bludau M, Kron F, et al. Profit center analysis of esophagectomy: Economical analysis of transthoracic esophagectomy depending on postoperative complications. Chirurg. 2018;89(3):229–36. [Article in German].
21. Nimptsch U, Krautz C, Weber GF, et al. Nationwide in-hospital mortality following pancreatic surgery in Germany is higher than anticipated. Ann Surg. 2016;264(6):1082–90.
22. Alsfasser G, Leicht H, Günster C, et al. Volume-outcome relationship in pancreatic surgery. Br J Surg. 2016;103(1):136–43.
23. Krautz C, Nimptsch U, Weber GF, et al. Effect of hospital volume on in-hospital morbidity and mortality following pancreatic surgery in Germany. Ann Surg. 2018;267(3):411–7.
24. Pieper D, Eikermann M, Mathes T, et al. Minimum thresholds under scrutiny. Chirurg. 2014;85(2):121–4. [Article in German].
25. Geraedts M, Kuhnen C, Cruppe W, Blum K, Ohmann C. Hospitals failing minimum volumes in 2004: reasons and consequences. Gesundheitswesen. 2008;70(2):63–7. [Article in German].
26. Krautz C, Denz A, Weber GF, Grutzmann R. Influence of hospital volume effects and minimum caseload requirements on quality of care in pancreatic surgery in Germany. Visc Med. 2017;33(2):131–4.

27. Balzano G, Zerbi A, Capretti G, et al. Effect of hospital volume on outcome of pancreaticoduodenectomy in Italy. Br J Surg. 2008;95(3):357–62.
28. Amato L, Fusco D, Acampora A, et al. Volume and health outcomes: evidence from systematic reviews and from evaluation of Italian hospital data. Epidemiol Prev. 2017;41(5–6 Suppl 2):1–128.
29. Bassi C. Surgery in Italy. Criteria to identify the hospital units and the tertiary referral centers entitled to perform it: a proposal for esophageal, hepatic, pancreatic and colo-rectal surgery. Updat Surg. 2016;68(2):115–6.
30. Parise P, Elmore U, Fumagalli U, et al. Esophageal surgery in Italy. Criteria to identify the hospital units and the tertiary referral centers entitled to perform it. Updat Surg. 2016;68(2):129–33.
31. Torzilli G, Viganò L, Giuliante F, Pinna AD. Liver surgery in Italy. Criteria to identify the hospital units and the tertiary referral centers entitled to perform it. Updat Surg. 2016;68(2):135–42.
32. Ruffo G, Barugola G, Rossini R, Sartori CA. Colorectal surgery in Italy. Criteria to identify the hospital units and the tertiary referral centers entitled to perform it. Updat Surg. 2016;68(2):123–8.
33. Stella M, Bissolati M, Gentile D, Arriciati A. Impact of surgical experience on management and outcome of pancreatic surgery performed in high- and low-volume centers. Updat Surg. 2017;69(3):351–8.
34. Lundstrom NR, Berggren H, Bjorkhem G, et al. Centralization of pediatric heart surgery in Sweden. Pediatr Cardiol. 2000;21(4):353–7.
35. Nymo LS, Soreide K, Kleive D, et al. The effect of centralization on short term outcomes of pancreatoduodenectomy in a universal health care system. HPB (Oxford). 2019;21(3):319–27.
36. Morales-García D. Towards the centralization of digestive oncologic surgery: changes in activity, techniques and outcome. Rev Esp Enferm Dig. 2017;110(1):65–6.
37. Manchon-Walsh P, Aliste L, Espinàs JA, et al. Improving survival and local control in rectal cancer in Catalonia (Spain) in the context of centralisation: a full cycle audit assessment. Eur J Surg Oncol. 2016;42(12):1873–80.
38. Ortiz H, Codina A, Ciga MA, et al. Effect of hospital caseload on long-term outcome after standardization of rectal cancer surgery in the Spanish Rectal Cancer Project. Cir Esp. 2016;94(8):442–52.
39. Gottlieb-Vedi E, Mattsson F, Lagergren P, Lagergren J. Annual hospital volume of surgery for gastrointestinal cancer in relation to prognosis. Eur J Surg Oncol. 2019;45(10):1839–46.
40. Derogar M, Blomberg J, Sadr-Azodi O. Hospital teaching status and volume related to mortality after pancreatic cancer surgery in a national cohort. Br J Surg. 2015;102(5):548–57.
41. Güller U, Warschkow R, Ackermann CJ, et al. Lower hospital volume is associated with higher mortality after oesophageal, gastric, pancreatic and rectal cancer resection. Swiss Med Wkly. 2017;147:w14473. https://doi.org/10.4414/smw.2017.14473.
42. Mesman R, Faber MJ, Berden B, Westert GP. Evaluation of minimum volume standards for surgery in the Netherlands (2003–2017): a successful policy? Health Policy. 2017;121(12):1263–73.
43. Svederud I, Virhage M, Medin E, et al. Patient perspectives on centralisation of low volume, highly specialised procedures in Sweden. Health Policy. 2015;119(8):1068–75.
44. Vallejo-Torres L, Melnychuk M, Vindrola-Padros C, et al. Discrete-choice experiment to analyse preferences for centralizing specialist cancer surgery services. Br J Surg. 2018;105(5):587–96.
45. Melnychuk M, Vindrola-Padros C, Aitchison M, et al. Centralising specialist cancer surgery services in England: survey of factors that matter to patients and carers and health professionals. BMC Cancer. 2018;18(1):226. https://doi.org/10.1186/s12885-018-4137-8.
46. Shalowitz DI, Nivasch E, Burger RA, Schapira MM. Are patients willing to travel for better ovarian cancer care? Gynecol Oncol. 2018;148(1):42–8.
47. Alvino DML, Chang DC, Adler JT, et al. How far are patients willing to travel for gastrectomy? Ann Surg. 2017;265(6):1172–7.
48. Smith AK, Shara NM, Zeymo A, et al. Travel patterns of cancer surgery patients in a regionalized system. J Surg Res. 2015;199(1):97–105.

49. Schlottmann F, Strassle PD, Charles AG, Patti MG. Esophageal cancer surgery: spontaneous centralization in the US contributed to reduce mortality without causing health disparities. Ann Surg Oncol. 2018;25(6):1580–7.
50. Cooke DT. Centralization of esophagectomy in the United States: might it benefit underserved populations? Ann Surg Oncol. 2018;25(6):1463–4.
51. Raoof M, Dumitra S, Ituarte PHG, et al. Centralization of pancreatic cancer surgery: travel distances and disparities. J Am Coll Surg. 2016;223(4 Suppl 2):e166. https://doi.org/10.1016/j.jamcollsurg.2016.08.422.
52. Mesman R, Faber MJ, Westert GP, Berden B. Exploring Dutch surgeons' views on volume-based policies: a qualitative interview study. J Health Serv Res Policy. 2018;23(3):185–92.
53. Greenberg CC, Ashley SW, Schrag D. Centralization of cancer surgery: what does it mean for surgical training? J Clin Oncol. 2009;27(28):4637–9.

Implications of the Relationship Between Volume and Performance in the USA

15

Jason B. Liu and Fabrizio Michelassi

15.1 Challenges in Studying Volume-Outcome Relationship

The earliest report of a volume-outcome relationship in surgery dates to the 1970s when Luft et al. [1] showed higher mortality rates in patients who underwent high-risk, complex operations at low-volume centers. Since then, hundreds of population-based studies have followed [2–5]. In the US, the most frequently cited volume-outcome studies have used large administrative datasets involving data from the Centers for Medicare and Medicaid Services (CMS), the National Inpatient Sample (NIS), and the Surveillance, Epidemiology, and End Results Program (SEER). In the aggregate, the studies have reaffirmed the correlation between surgical volume and outcomes to varying degrees across multiple surgical specialties and operations. However, no national policy exists mandating volume minimums for hospitals or surgeons because all these studies face several challenges [6–8].

First, although the volume-outcome association is relatively simple to investigate when it comes to operative volume and patient mortality, this correlation has been usually limited to within the hospital stay or 30 days postoperatively, a limited time horizon. Furthermore, complications, length of stay, readmission, reoperation, discharge destination, postoperative functional status, patient satisfaction, and long-term outcomes may be more appropriate variables to study this correlation. Very few studies have examined whether the volume-outcome association extends to these other outcomes or over longer time periods.

J. B. Liu
Department of Surgery, University of Chicago Medicine, Chicago, IL, USA
e-mail: Jason.Liu@uchospitals.edu

F. Michelassi (✉)
Department of Surgery, New York-Presbyterian Hospital at Weill Cornell,
New York, NY, USA
e-mail: fam2006@med.cornell.edu

© Springer Nature Switzerland AG 2021
M. Montorsi (ed.), *Volume-Outcome Relationship in Oncological Surgery*,
Updates in Surgery, https://doi.org/10.1007/978-3-030-51806-6_15

A second challenge is posed by the absence of clear agreement on "low" versus "high" volume centers. Volume thresholds are set arbitrarily because no study has been able to rigorously determine precise volume thresholds above which outcomes clearly and causally change. Ravi et al. [9] conducted a cohort study in Canada that revealed a minimum annual threshold of 35 total hip arthroplasties per surgeon to decrease the risk of dislocation and revision. Using identical methods, Adam et al. [10] identified a surgeon volume threshold of 25 annual thyroidectomies that was associated with improved patient outcomes. Unfortunately, both studies utilized a methodology that is not statistically robust; and, no thresholds have been identified at the hospital level [11, 12]. Volume thresholds in different studies are based on administrative data, expert panels, percentiles, or literature review and may differ not only from study to study but also from operation to operation. For example, when LaPar et al. [13] analyzed volume as a continuous variable, they identified no volume-outcome relationship. It is likely that a volume-outcome relationship is mathematically asymptotic and does not inherently include an inflection point.

A third challenge is represented by the fact that the volume-outcome relationship, well-established in the aggregate at a hospital level, does not maintain its relationship at the individual surgeon level. In other words, there may be surgeons with low volume and good results and surgeons with high volumes and consistently higher morbidity and mortality. This hypothesis is difficult to analyze due to the low statistical power of small numbers. It is surmised that low volume surgeons may have excellent outcomes because of experience or because they perform a high volume of similar operations requiring similar technical skills [14].

15.2 Challenges in Centralizing Surgical Care in the USA

Despite these challenges, the abundant literature in favor of the volume-outcome relationship has spurred an interest in centralization (or regionalization) of surgical care in the US. Consideration to regionalize certain high-risk operations did not occur until the Institute of Medicine (IOM) report in 1999 sparked the formation of the Leapfrog Group, a conglomerate of businesses that sought better healthcare transparency for their employees. This healthcare watchdog organization initially set volume standards for five high-risk procedures and has now expanded to eight procedures with volume thresholds for both hospitals and surgeons [15].

Recently, the "Take the Volume Pledge" campaign, led by Dartmouth-Hitchcock Medical Center, the Johns Hopkins Hospital and Health System, and the University of Michigan Health System, reignited the volume standard debate after being publicly announced on May 18, 2015 in *U.S. News & World Report* [16]. Yet, a recent article [17] has found that the Leapfrog Group's minimum volume standards did not differentiate hospitals based on mortality for three high-risk cancer operations assessed (esophageal, lung and rectal resections) at hospitals meeting the volume standards, with mortality rates consistently lower only after pancreatic resections.

Although commendable, mandating that certain operations are performed only in high-volume centers has consequences for patients, families and providers.

Patients and families may be exposed to increased travel distance and time, increased cost of travel, prolonged wait times, inability to seek local emergency care, limited access to routine surgical care, and fragmentation of the continuity of care when complications from a complex operation arise. Several key studies have examined the burden of increased travel distance and time on patients referred to high-volume centers [18, 19]. In addition, obtaining care near home is of particular importance to many patients, especially as they age. For example, Liu et al. [20] demonstrated that driving distance in rural locations likely remains the main reason why patients choose to undergo complex cancer operations at a low-volume center. Studies examining other consequences and ramifications to patients are ongoing. No study to date has comprehensively examined patient referral patterns or surveyed patient decision-making [21].

A policy of centralization may also have consequences on the surgeons, surgical teams and hospitals [22]. As more patients are referred to high-volume centers, resources of high-volume centers may become stressed and resources to low-volume hospitals in the more isolated and underserved areas may be further depleted. In addition, surgeons may become inadequately prepared to perform complex operations in emergent situations, or they may even become unfamiliar with complications from complex operations performed at high-volume hospitals. These unintended consequences need to be considered when considering health policies that regionalize healthcare in the US.

15.3   The Role of the American College of Surgeons

In recognition of these challenges, the American College of Surgeons (ACS) created a task force in 2015 to reexamine the contemporary relationship between volume and outcomes in order to give guidance in terms of credentialing and privileges for surgeons. The task force reviewed the literature on the subject and wrote a statement, which was approved by the ACS Board of Regents at their meeting in February 2018 and published online on April 1, 2018 [23]. An excerpt from the statement is worth reproducing: "For some 'complex' procedures, published evidence suggests that a high case volume is associated with improved surgical outcomes. However, these outcomes may reflect not only the knowledge, experience, and skill of the individual surgeon, but also the aggregate ability of the institution and hospital staff to provide high quality care for specific groups of patients. Thus, while high case volume of a particular 'complex' procedure is usually associated with better surgical outcomes, these two are not synonymous. It is well documented that some surgeons performing a relatively low volume of the procedure also achieve excellent outcomes" [23].

Currently, the ACS is in the process of creating several manuals for optimal resources for high-risk, complex operations (gastrointestinal surgery, thoracic surgery, vascular surgery, emergency general surgery) to add to the already existing manuals for trauma, cancer, pediatrics, and geriatrics. This movement is in recognition that, independent of volume, the safety and quality of surgical procedures depend on surgeon and professional staff training, surgeon experience and skills, the available institutional resources, and the ability to validly measure surgical outcomes. These manuals offer standards for structures, resources and processes of care, which can be measured for continuous quality improvement.

15.4   Centralization Trends in the US Hospitals

Although the US does not have policies that centralize surgical care, there are emerging data that high-risk procedures are done less and less frequently at low-volume hospitals [17]. In a recent study on pancreatoduodenectomies (PD) in New York, Florida and California from 2002 through 2012, there was a decrease in the number of low-volume centers and an increase in the number of higher-volume centers performing PD [24]. In fact, a high number of low-volume centers stopped performing PD cases altogether over the study period. This and other studies support the statement that centralization of high-risk procedures is occurring in the US. This was well demonstrated by a similar study in Washington State with the intent of documenting "migration" of more complex operations from low- to higher-volume centers [25]. The authors analyzed three operations (pancreatectomy, esophagectomy, and abdominal aortic aneurysm repair) in all 65 hospitals in Washington State for the 7 years before and 7 years after the Leapfrog recommendations. The authors demonstrated that migration occurred in 80% of those cases done in high volume hospitals by the end of the study. The study also identified that the patients that did not "migrate" were poorer and had higher comorbidities, thus yielding a higher mortality in the hospitals where they had to stay. The authors concluded that the migration did not improve results overall when mortality was viewed across the entire state.

Importantly, centralization in the US is occurring at a speed that is sensitive to many other considerations (e.g., population access and preference, financial and coverage issues, existing capacity in high-volume hospitals) rather than by fiat. Anecdotally, surgeons in low-volume hospitals are doing as much as they can to direct high-risk, complex operations to high-volume centers regardless of external impositions and, at the same time, they find themselves caring for high-risk patients because of patient's preferences or other constraining circumstances.

15.5   Conclusions

Improvements are certainly needed. It is likely that in the near future the American College of Surgeons will indicate a minimum number of high-risk cases to be performed in order to maintain verification in its quality programs. It may also be that in the future payers may use different tactics to steer patients to high-volume centers. Yet, it is likely that the ultimate solution for the US will be a balance between centralization of high-risk procedures to high-volume centers and nationwide improvement of the structures, resources and processes of care at low-volume centers, where a large percentage of the US population still receives surgical care.

References

1. Luft HS, Bunker JB, Enthoven AC. Should operations be regionalized? The empirical relation between surgical volume and mortality. N Engl J Med. 1979;301(25):1364–9.
2. Birkmeyer JD, Siewers AE, Finlayson EV, et al. Hospital volume and surgical mortality in the United States. N Engl J Med. 2002;346(15):1128–37.
3. Birkmeyer JD, Stukel TA, Siewers AE, et al. Surgeon volume and operative mortality in the United States. N Engl J Med. 2003;349(22):2117–27.
4. Finks JF, Osborne NH, Birkmeyer JD. Trends in hospital volume and operative mortality for high-risk surgery. N Engl J Med. 2011;364(22):2128–37.
5. Liu JH, Zingmond DS, McGory ML, et al. Disparities in the utilization of high-volume hospitals for complex surgery. JAMA. 2006;296(16):1973–80.
6. Khuri SF, Henderson WG. The case against volume as a measure of quality of surgical care. World J Surg. 2005;29(10):1222–9.
7. Russell TR. Invited commentary: volume standards for high-risk operations: an American College of Surgeons' view. Surgery. 2001;130(3):423–4.
8. Shahian DM, Normand SL. The volume-outcome relationship: from Luft to Leapfrog. Ann Thorac Surg. 2003;75(3):1048–58.
9. Ravi B, Jenkinson R, Austin PC, et al. Relation between surgeon volume and risk of complications after total hip arthroplasty: propensity score matched cohort study. BMJ. 2014;348:g3284. https://doi.org/10.1136/bmj.g3284.
10. Adam MA, Thomas S, Youngwirth L, et al. Is there a minimum number of thyroidectomies a surgeon should perform to optimize patient outcomes? Ann Surg. 2017;265(2):402–7.
11. Elixhauser A, Steiner C, Fraser I. Volume thresholds and hospital characteristics in the United States. Health Aff (Millwood). 2003;22(2):167–77.
12. Halm EA, Lee C, Chassin MR. Is volume related to outcome in health care? A systematic review and methodologic critique of the literature. Ann Intern Med. 2002;137(6):511–20.
13. LaPar DJ, Kron IL, Jones DR, et al. Hospital procedure volume should not be used as a measure of surgical quality. Ann Surg. 2012;256(4):606–15.
14. Urbach DR, Baxter NN. Does it matter what a hospital is "high volume" for? Specificity of hospital volume-outcome associations for surgical procedures: analysis of administrative data. BMJ. 2004;328(7442):737–40.
15. The Leapfrog Group. Surgical Volume. 2019. https://www.leapfroggroup.org/ratings-reports/surgical-volume. Accessed 30 Apr 2020.
16. Urbach DR. Pledging to eliminate low-volume surgery. N Engl J Med. 2015;373(15):1388–90.
17. Sheetz KH, Chhabra KR, Smith ME, et al. Association of discretionary hospital volume standards for high-risk cancer surgery with patient outcomes and access, 2005–2016. JAMA Surg. 2019;154(11):1005–12.
18. Dudley RA, Johansen KL, Brand R, et al. Selective referral to high-volume hospitals: estimating potentially avoidable deaths. JAMA. 2000;283(9):1159–66.
19. Birkmeyer JD, Siewers AE, Marth NJ, Goodman DC. Regionalization of high-risk surgery and implications for patient travel times. JAMA. 2003;290(20):2703–8.
20. Liu JB, Bilimoria KY, Mallin K, Winchester DP. Patient characteristics associated with undergoing cancer operations at low-volume hospitals. Surgery. 2017;161(2):433–43.
21. Finlayson SR, Birkmeyer JD, Tosteson AN, Nease RF Jr. Patient preferences for location of care: implications for regionalization. Med Care. 1999;37(2):204–9.
22. Schwartz DM, Fong ZV, Warshaw AL, et al. The hidden consequences of the volume pledge: "no patient left behind"? Ann Surg. 2017;265(2):273–4.
23. American College of Surgeons. Statement on credentialing and privileging and volume performance issues. 2018. https://www.facs.org/about-acs/statements/111-credentialing. Accessed 30 Apr 2020.
24. O'Mahoney PRA, Yeo HL, Sedrakyan A, et al. Centralization of pancreatoduodenectomy a decade later: impact of the volume-outcome relationship. Surgery. 2016;159(6):1528–38.
25. Massarweh NN, Flum DR, Symons RG, et al. A critical evaluation of the impact of Leapfrog's evidence-based hospital referral. J Am Coll Surg. 2011;212(2):150–9.e1.

Assistance to Cancer Patients: Their Point of View

16

Antonio Gaudioso, Valeria Fava, and Tiziana Nicoletti

16.1 Civic Engagement and Health Promotion in Italy

Cittadinanzattiva is a movement of civic engagement established in 1978 and operating both in Italy and in Europe in the protection of human rights, the promotion and exercise of civil, social and political rights of citizens, and support for individuals who need help.

Our mission is related to the last paragraph of Article 118 of the Constitution of the Italian Republic, integrated in the 2001 constitutional reform. Article 118 recognizes the autonomous initiative of citizens, both individually and associated, in carrying out activities of general interest and, based on the principle of subsidiarity, requires the institutions to favor active citizens.

Our role is to report deficiencies, abuses, and non-fulfilments and act to prevent these from happening again through changes in society and behavior, as well as through the promotion of new policies and the implementation of laws and regulations. We believe that "acting as a citizen is the best way to be one", or better, that the action of citizens aware of their powers and responsibilities is a way to strengthen our democracy, protect our rights and promote the daily care of our common heritage.

Our objectives are to:

- empower citizens to participate in public policies by enhancing their skills and their point of view;
- protect citizens by preventing injustices and unnecessary suffering;
- inform and change behaviors harmful to the general interest;

A. Gaudioso (✉) · V. Fava · T. Nicoletti
Cittadinanzattiva onlus, Rome, Italy
e-mail: a.gaudioso@cittadinanzattiva.it; v.fava@cittadinanzattiva.it;
t.nicoletti@cittadinanzattiva.it

© Springer Nature Switzerland AG 2021
M. Montorsi (ed.), *Volume-Outcome Relationship in Oncological Surgery*,
Updates in Surgery, https://doi.org/10.1007/978-3-030-51806-6_16

- implement the rights recognized by the law and favor the recognition of new rights;
- protect and take care of our common heritage;
- provide citizens with the appropriate tools in order to take action and communicate at a more informed level with the institutions;
- build alliances and collaborations necessary to resolve conflicts and promote rights.

In particular, Cittadinanzattiva—with its networks, such as the Tribunal for Patients' Rights and the National Coordination of Chronic Patients' Associations—protects and promotes the rights of citizens in health and welfare services with the aim of contributing to a more humane, effective and rational organization of the National Health Service.

16.1.1 Tribunal for Patients' Rights

The Tribunal for Patients' Rights (TDM, Tribunale per i diritti del malato) is an initiative of Cittadinanzattiva, established in 1980, to protect and promote the rights of citizens in health and welfare services and to contribute to a more humane, effective and rational organization of the National Health Service. The TDM is a network made up of ordinary citizens, but also of operators from a wide range of services as well as of professionals who commit on a voluntary basis (ca. 10,000).

We operate through:

- about 300 local offices, covering all of Italy, in hospitals and local services;
- a central organization which coordinates the network's activities and promotes national initiatives;
- national, regional and local thematic groups, linked to specific programs;
- regional coordination, support for local networks and for the promotion of regional policies for the protection of health rights;
- an integrated health protection project (PiT Salute, Progetto integrato di tutela della salute), providing information, consultancy and assistance for citizens on health and social services, active at national, regional and local levels; the PiT Salute services collect around 25,000 reports each year, which have been processed and published in the annual *Rapporto PiT Salute* since 1997.

The activities of the TDM are aimed at finding solutions to eliminate unnecessary suffering and injustice, organizing public protests and resorting to the judicial authority, thus favoring the exercise of the powers to understand each situation, mobilizing consciences, redressing institutional setbacks, and finally achieving as promptly as possible concrete changes in order to amend rights which have been violated. Integral parts of the TDM activities are the promotion and implementation of policies aimed at asserting the point of view of citizens in the reform of health welfare.

As part of its overall objectives in contributing to the improvement, quality and humanization of health services, TDM's key objectives are:

- to guarantee that when citizens need assistance, advice or help in asserting their legitimate expectations, they have both the tools and the opportunities to obtain the protection of their rights;
- to promote civic engagement, so that citizens themselves are actors in the forefront for the protection of their health rights, both through TDM and through civic engagement in the health sector.

16.1.2 National Coordination of Chronic Patients' Associations

The National Coordination of Chronic Patients' Associations (CnAMC, Coordinamento Nazionale delle Associazioni dei Malati Cronici) is a network of Cittadinanzattiva established in 1996, and is an example of a transversal alliance between Associations and Federations of people suffering from chronic and rare diseases for the protection of their rights. It defines and pursues common social and health policies based on an integrated and coherent protection; it acts as a platform for requests and proposals forwarded by associations; it favors the exchange of positive experiences also among organizations; it organizes training programs for the growth of leadership. The CnAMC has currently more than 100 member associations. Every year it produces a National Report about the policies of the Chronic Care Act to focus attention on the many critical issues of public health care of people with chronic and rare diseases and their impact on their families. The Report is a platform based on the requests, expectations and proposals of the Associations which are part of the CnAMC and aims at overcoming any difficulties encountered. Moreover, it is implemented through the participation and active collaboration of Patient Associations which provide information on the recommendations forwarded by its members and on the experiences of citizens' care programs.

16.1.3 Our Commitment to Protecting Cancer Patients

Cittadinanzattiva has been continuously promoting for several years now projects, information and awareness-raising campaigns for people with cancer, and is committed to strengthening the power of intervention of citizens in public policies through empowerment and making their voices heard, by collecting and disseminating good practices, evaluating services and providing civic information (surveys and civic monitoring), as well as promoting ad hoc assistance policies.

One of the distinctive features of Cittadinanzattiva's work has always been the implementation of actions aimed at promoting cultural change and the creation of collaborations and synergies, involving all actors, from patient associations and healthcare professionals, to health companies and institutional representatives.

Our objective is to network, share good practices, identify and better focus on problems, solutions and proposals in order to improve the quality of care and encourage the empowerment of individual and associated citizens.

Regarding cancer, over the years we have promoted several activities such as:

- a survey on home-based cancer care and the fight against unnecessary pain;
- campaigns for empowerment;
- protection of citizens' rights;
- promotion of good practices through the Andrea Alesini Award;
- civic audits;
- the civic observatory on federalism in health;
- civic monitoring of oncological centers [1];
- reports on various topics of the service provided by National Health System, such as the personalization of care, respect for time, and informed consent in oncology [2] and the organization of hematology-oncology day units [3];
- the recent exploratory pilot survey on the services for genetic tests [4].

16.2   Challenges for the Future

The incidence of tumors in the Italian population is high, although it has shown a decline in the last period: the estimate for 2019 is 371,000 diagnoses (196,000 men and 175,000 women), as against 373,000 in 2018, equal to a decline of 2000 in 12 months [5]. Epidemiological data show a trend to be considered: around 1000 people are diagnosed with cancer every day; this is a significant number that underlines the burden of oncological diseases and the continuous effort to improve the survival rate of patients not only in quantitative terms, but also in terms of quality of life.

In fact, medicine and research have identified increasingly effective tools and actions aimed at each unique case, from prevention and early diagnosis to therapy, in order to improve the prognosis for each person in terms of survival. Nowadays, new diagnostic methods are rapidly revolutionizing the therapeutic approach to cancer, based on molecular analyses together with the interpretation of big data and the availability of new drugs. Data from the genetic profile of a patient's tumor can now be analyzed in order to offer the most suitable therapy for that specific patient at that time, in a process known as personalized medicine. The term "personalized medicine" has its own specific meaning indicating, beyond individual genomic characteristics, a methodology that provides an overall evaluation incorporating other individual characteristics, such as gender, ethnicity, lifestyle and comorbidity, in order to qualitatively, quantitatively and in terms of time adapt prevention, diagnosis or therapy according to the single patient's needs. Treating a patient increasingly means taking care of that patient, with his or her characteristics and individual response to drugs, with everything that makes him or her unique even though suffering from a disease common with others.

Another rapidly developing area is genetic testing. An example is the BRCA test. Adoption of the BRCA genetic test in the prevention and treatment of breast and ovarian cancer began almost 20 years ago, soon after doctors started to understand its importance. Thanks to clinical research carried out by several research institutes and universities, the BRCA test became immediately available in Italy and several centers throughout the country have been efficiently offering it since then. This marked the beginning of a new branch of medicine was born, referred to as "oncological genetics" or "oncogenetics", which brings together the skills of the geneticist and those of the oncologist in order to foster new knowledge on the hereditary predisposition to tumors in clinical practice, both for patients with hereditary cancer and for healthy subjects who are at greater risk of cancer since they are genetically predisposed. In recent years there has been a rapid expansion of the use of the BRCA test which has not been accompanied by an increase in the health system's capacity to train experienced professionals in the sector. The difficulty of transferring the necessary expertise to a large number of professionals regarding a new, little known and rapidly evolving field has affected all countries, not just Italy.

Besides in-depth knowledge and the best diagnostic and therapeutic opportunities, what is always important is the overall care of the patient, and early recognition of his or her physical, functional, social, psychological and rehabilitative needs, prevention and control of symptoms related to the disease or therapies, as well as the relevance of care, all issues that will need to be tackled in the near future.

Today oncologic diseases are becoming increasingly "chronic" since more and more people are affected, so that great efforts must be made to improve their quality of life. Taking care of patients means guaranteeing a systemic pathway, one that is accessible, timely, and attentive to individual needs and to the context in which the patient lives.

16.3 Priorities for Cancer Patients

From the data collected, the critical points and difficulties for a patient suffering from cancer are considerable. Our latest survey of the issues related to cancer patients shows an analysis of data from the PiT Salute daily reports and from the headquarters of the Tribunal for Patients' Rights of Cittadinanzattiva as well as an analysis of data from oncology monitoring carried out on 63 oncology centers, 46 oncology day hospitals and about 1000 patient interviews. The data analyzed allowed us to trace the level of care to cancer patients through the strengths and weaknesses of our health system.

In the survey we followed the progress of a cancer patient through access to services for diagnosis and treatment, how the centers managed the patient by guaranteeing a multidisciplinary approach, directing him to the currently available services, helping with paperwork and with the transition from hospital to home, while ensuring respect of the individual, his psychological needs and personalization of care.

The *XXI Rapporto PiT Salute* [6] highlights a number of sensitive issues for the year 2017:

* long waiting lists for cancer surgery: 13.2%;
* long waiting lists for specialist visits: 9.9% with about an 8-month waiting list;
* long waiting lists for diagnostic tests: 16.8%;
* long waiting lists for chemotherapy and radiotherapy: 10%;
* access to drugs: 10.7%;
* healthcare mobility: oncology ranks first with a relative figure of 38.7% of the total;
* difficulties regarding hospital care: 19.2%.

The first problem regards access to diagnostic, therapeutic and surgical operations related to cancer. Over one in ten citizens who contact us report long waiting lists for diagnostic tests (e.g., on average 13 months for a mammography and 9 months for a colonoscopy) and for surgery. The percentage of citizens with long waiting lists for specialist visits (about 8 months on average) and also for chemo- and radiotherapy is slightly lower (10%). Waiting lists are not guaranteed everywhere, even in the case of emergencies: about one-fourth complain of having waited to access diagnostic and specialist services in the case of diagnostic suspicion more than the 72 h set by the National Plan on waiting lists [7], and about 13%, after the diagnosis, waited for more than 60 days for surgery. Regarding how quick a diagnosis is made, Italy has further critical issues related to prevention through organized screening programs. The latest report on the Coordination of Public Finance 2018 shows a persistent significant geographical discrepancy. As a rating of 9 is considered a satisfactory assessment (defining a Region fulfilling all prevention actions set by the Essential Levels of Care), there are five Regions that do not reach acceptable ratings: Calabria (2) Puglia (4), Campania and Sicily (3), and Sardinia (5) against a rating of 15 for Valle D'Aosta and Veneto. The reason for these differences are manifold (cultural, organizational, accessibility to services, etc.), but one of the most important is undoubtedly that of "active calls", i.e., informing the target population, which is ineffective in many Regions of southern Italy and is not able to reach every citizen.

Regarding access to drugs, although most of the monitored facilities (42%) respond that on average the inclusion of new drugs in the hospital formulary (the list of drugs actually available to patients) is almost immediate (0–15 days), in many cases it can also take several months: 7% from 3 to 4 months and 9% from 4 to 6 months. The same must be said for the inclusion of so-called innovative drugs in the formulary: on average 60% are available after 1 month, more than a quarter after 2 months, and 2% after more than 6 months. The reason for this is almost always Italian excessive red tape regarding access to medicines, so effective provision of drugs to patients goes through too many, often redundant, phases that inevitably extend supply times. Another consideration is related to the costs of therapies for innovative cancer drugs that often affect the budgets of regional and hospital medicine supplies. Therefore, the Italian Budget Law has allocated, through the 2017, a fund of one billion euros to be distributed to the Regions in order to allow more widespread access to innovative therapies.

As for accepting a patient immediately after a diagnosis, 90% of facilities act promptly and 50% assign the 048 exemption code, a code provided in Italy to guarantee free diagnosis and treatment of cancer.

Eighty-nine percent of the centers monitored guarantee a multidisciplinary team in case management, ensuring participation of all specialists directly involved in the therapeutic diagnostic pathway. Nonetheless, there are a series of inconsistencies, i.e., not always being able to guarantee some professional key figures in the multidisciplinary team: in 80% of cases a social worker and the family doctor are missing, in 66% the nutritionist, in 55% the pain therapist or palliative care specialist, in 38% the psychologist. Also case managers are guaranteed in only one in three centers.

Regarding patient assistance, the time and quality of information received during the first visit is a sore point: about one person in four considers the information and the time reserved just about sufficient or inadequate. About one-third say that they have not received an appointment for further consultations or investigations required by the specialist, but have to go back to the general practitioner for a prescription or book an appointment independently through a booking center. In one day-hospital out of five there is no phone service to report emergencies, problems caused by the therapy or to ask for advice, so patients have to refer to the Emergency Department.

After being discharged from hospital, more than one citizen out of four complains about the lack of responsiveness at community level, in part because just over one-third of facilities have a person to refer to who can continue to provide care.

Regarding humanization of care, although most of the facilities monitored claim to guarantee attention to pain as required by Law 38/2010 [8] as well as personalized care, 75% of patients do not immediately carry out psychological assessments and 66% do not provide programs to protect the reproductive function in cancer patients. Furthermore, in helping patients with red tape, 40% of citizens complain of lack of support in administrative procedures, e.g., for the issuing of prostheses and aids, or certification of civil disability and handicap or co-payment exemptions.

Those who are struggling with cancer, whether patients or family/friends caring for them (caregivers), bear a considerable burden both economically and in terms of time.

Work-care relationships are affected by considerable stress and changes for both patients and caregivers: both have to reorganize their lifestyles to adapt to new schedules and rhythms, as well as to more demanding health needs. Both patients and caregivers have often to give up work during the treatment, with all the resulting consequences, economic and other.

Sixty-eight percent of patients interviewed as part of our monitoring program need the assistance, for example for day hospital therapy, of a family member, who works in 56% of cases. This clearly shows the impact the time spent inside the day hospital has on the life of both patients and families. Patients and family members tell us of the many difficulties they have in adjusting the rhythms of daily life to the need for care, asking for treatment permits, having to give up free time activities in order to be able to care for or support one's loved one in a moment of need.

In many cases people feel they are just numbers on a list, a bed, and not human beings with their own dignity, feelings and personal history. There is still too little training and selection of personnel for patient management, not only from a clinical point of view, but also from a human one. Personalized medicine and the humanization of care are the two challenges for the future. We need to adapt medical care to people's needs, which are many and varied, especially in the more internal areas and in our cities, in order to guarantee transparent access to innovation and a program of humanization of care which includes also the needs of people, as well as quick accesses and organization of services as befits a civil and civilized country.

Setting up oncology networks is a further challenge. Oncology networks are defined by the Ministry of Health as "the best model for oncology" but are active in only a few Italian Regions: Piedmont and Valle d'Aosta, Lombardy, Veneto, Tuscany, Umbria, Liguria, the autonomous Province of Trento, Puglia and Campania.

The Reviewed Organizational Guidelines and Recommendations for the Oncology Network, which integrates acute and post-acute hospital care with community programs, envisages a series of key points, guaranteeing equity of access to care and early admission to care, based on epidemiological evidence, analysis of needs and of the population; understanding all the parts in the network; being consistent with national accreditation and hospital standards. We strongly believe that a key point for a humanized approach to the care of cancer patients is to support them by managing and solving all bureaucratic barriers (unjustified long waiting lists for booking tests and/or visits, carrying out diagnostic-therapeutic procedures, collecting medical reports, etc.), making life easier and allowing patients to face their upcoming treatment.

The regional cancer network, which we hope will be implemented for patient management and which will necessarily have to connect to other regional networks, must serve as a bridge for continuity of care between the hospital and the community, an organizational model with a multidisciplinary approach integrating specialist care with a "specialized cancer team" for the clinical management of patients, sharing care programs and guaranteeing fair access to treatment and an early admission to hospital.

The perspective is precisely that of a health system based on the principles of efficiency, effectiveness, quality and safety which must first of all create programs to manage all the phases of the disease in the most appropriate way: those that require hospitalization in special high-complexity referral centers; those that require hospitalization in less complex centers, or treatments carried out at the patient's home with the family doctor, with consequent significant psychological and practical advantages for the patient.

References

1. Gaudioso A. Vincoli e aspettative dei pazienti [Patients' constraints and expectations]. Presentation to Cancer Real World 2019 "From needs to challenges". Milan, 24–25 January 2019. http://www.chrp.it/wp-content/uploads/1040_Gaudioso.pdf. Accessed 30 Apr 2020.
2. Cittadinanzattiva. Oncologia: personalizzazione delle cure, rispetto del tempo, consenso informato. Focus sul cancro del colon retto [Oncology: personalization of care, respect for time, and informed consent. Focus on colorectal cancer]. Rome. 2012. https://www.quotidianosanita.it/allegati/allegato8196654.pdf. Accessed 30 Apr 2020.
3. Cittadinanzattiva. Monitoraggio civico dei day hospital onco-ematologici [Civic monitoring of oncology-hematology day hospitals]. Rome. 2019. https://sostieni.cittadinanzattiva.it/scarica-i-materiali/monitoraggio-civico-dei-day-hospital-onco-ematologici/viewdocument.html. Accessed 30 Apr 2020.
4. Cittadinanzattiva. Test genetici: tra prevenzione e diritto alle cure. Focus BRCA [Genetic tests: between prevention and right to treatment. Focus on BRCA]. Rome. 2019. https://cittadinanzattiva.it/files/progetti/salute/Report_BRCA_Final_Sito_CA.pdf. Accessed 30 Apr 2020.
5. AIOM (Associazione Italiana di Oncologia Medica) and AIRTUM (Associazione Italiana dei Registri Tumori). I numeri del cancro in Italia 2019 [Cancer figures in Italy 2019]. https://www.aiom.it/wp-content/uploads/2019/09/2019_Numeri_Cancro-operatori-web.pdf. Accessed 30 Apr 2020.
6. Cittadinanzattiva. XXI Rapporto PiT Salute. Tra attese e costi, il futuro della salute in gioco [Between waiting times and costs, the future of health at stake]. https://www.quotidianosanita.it/allegati/allegato2745424.pdf. Accessed 30 Apr 2020.
7. Ministero della Salute. Piano nazionale di governo delle liste di attesa per il triennio 2019–2021 [Ministry of Health. National waiting list governance plan for years 2019–2021]. http://www.salute.gov.it/portale/listeAttesa/dettaglioPubblicazioniListeAttesa.jsp?lingua=italiano&id=2824.
8. Legge 15 marzo 2010, n. 38. Disposizioni per garantire l'accesso alle cure palliative e alla terapia del dolore [Law March 15, 2010, n. 38. Provisions to ensure access to palliative care and pain therapy]. https://www.gazzettaufficiale.it/gunewsletter/dettaglio.jsp?service=1&data gu=2010-03-19&task=dettaglio&numgu=65&redaz=010G0056&tmstp=1269600292070.

Centralization and the Accreditation Process: A Mutual Relationship

Matteo Donadon, Grazia Maria Attinà, Elena Vanni,
Pierluigi Marini, and Marco Montorsi

17.1 Introduction

In the previous chapters of this book, some of the world-wide experts on different fields of surgical oncology addressed the significance of the volume-outcome relationship, highlighting what is good and what is less good in such a union. While some conclusions are data-driven and straightforward, others are extrapolated and more complicated to be translated into clinical practice. As previously stated, in the context of different health systems worldwide, from national health systems to private insurances, there are different stakeholders—politicians, patients, surgeons, institutions and medical associations—whose needs do not always match. Moreover, clinicians and organizations have to find a balance between the demand for high-quality surgery and the current inadequate reimbursements for most of the general

M. Donadon
Department of Biomedical Sciences, Humanitas University, Pieve Emanuele, Milan, Italy
Department of Hepatobiliary and General Surgery,
Humanitas Clinical and Research Center IRCCS, Rozzano, Milan, Italy
e-mail: matteo.donadon@hunimed.eu

G. M. Attinà · P. Marini
Department of General Surgery, S. Camillo-Forlanini Hospital, Rome, Italy
e-mail: graziamaria.attina@gmail.com; pmarini@scamilloforlanini.rm.it

E. Vanni
Business Operations, Humanitas Clinical and Research Center IRCCS, Rozzano, Milan, Italy
e-mail: elena.vanni@humanitas.it

M. Montorsi (✉)
Department of Biomedical Sciences, Humanitas University, Pieve Emanuele, Milan, Italy
Department of General Surgery, Humanitas Clinical and Research Center IRCCS, Rozzano, Milan, Italy
e-mail: marco.montorsi@hunimed.eu

© Springer Nature Switzerland AG 2021   177
M. Montorsi (ed.), *Volume-Outcome Relationship in Oncological Surgery*,
Updates in Surgery, https://doi.org/10.1007/978-3-030-51806-6_17

oncological surgical procedures which, together with the contraction of public funding for the Italian National Health System (NHS), make it difficult to implement quality. Starting from case studies of the reimbursements for hepatopancreatobiliary (HPB) surgery and colorectal cancer (CRC) surgery, this last chapter will focus on some important issues including the accreditation process and put forward some practical proposals that will hopefully serve as a constructive action plan.

17.2   NHS Reimbursements: Case Studies on HPB Surgery

The high-quality care granted by high surgical volume, coupled with the ability to measure clinical outcomes, is the direct consequence of a system of care [1]. However, the system of care implies that all types of resources, including facilities, services, health professionals as well as organization administration and managers, should be dedicated to only a few specialized subjects and should cover all the phases of the care cycle. In this sense, the reimbursement system should take into consideration not only the caseload but also the quality of care. Unfortunately, the reimbursement system in Italy does not consider the quality of the results.

Italian hospitals are currently reimbursed according to some discharge fees that are based on the diagnosis-related group codes (DRG–ICD-9-CM, version 24). The current coding system does not separate hepatobiliary from pancreatic procedures, and only one code is available. Table 17.1 shows the current values for HPB surgery in Italy. As is known, there are two types of reimbursements depending on the presence of complications, with the NHS providing a larger reimbursement in cases with complications. However, when comparing these values with the actual resources absorbed in the care process, it is evident that the reimbursement system should be revised. Notably, these resources may be divided into those which absorb hospital assets (i.e., beds, operating rooms, equipment and in general all the other finite resources) and those generally considered running costs (i.e., drugs and materials). The first resources are limited since they are in competition with other hospital units, while the second do not have an impact on the availability of physical or scarce resources. As detailed in Table 17.1, the estimated average costs for a single inpatient episode of HPB surgery, either with or without complications, exceed the

Table 17.1 Current values and costs for HPB surgery at the Humanitas Clinical and Research Center

		Reimbursement[a]	Average costs[b]	Delta
Pancreas, liver, and shunt procedures	With complications[c]	18,833 €	21,535 €	–2702 €
	Without complications[c]	7549 €	11,326 €	–3777 €

HPB hepatopancreatobiliary
[a]Values for a single episode of inpatient HPB surgery according to the DRG-ICD-9-CM, version 24
[b]Average of real costs of 1 year of episodes as calculated by the Office for Management Control
[c]Complications mean the presence of a secondary diagnosis of a condition that was present when the patient was admitted to the hospital (comorbidity) or one that developed during the hospitalization (postoperative complication)

amount reimbursed. Intriguingly, the costs are not simulated, being expressed as the average of real costs of 1 year of episodes as calculated by the Office for Management Control of Humanitas Clinical and Research Center—IRCCS (*unpublished data*). In contrast to HPB surgery, the Italian situation for CRC surgery is different. Indeed, considering that the running costs in CRC surgery are usually lower than in the case of HPB surgery, in which the use of albumin, expensive antibiotics and blood components is more common, and considering also that the amount of the reimbursements for laparotomic and/or laparoscopic colectomy are much more balanced, it follows that most HPB surgery is currently operating at a loss, while most CRC surgery is operating at least at the break-even point (*data unshown*).

The unsuitability and insufficiency of the current NHS reimbursements is even more evident when considering the application of new innovative surgical procedures. In CRC surgery, the application of the novel approach named Transanal Total Mesorectal Excision, which has emerged as an alternative to the traditional abdominal approach for rectal cancer, is associated with a significant cost increase of approximately €1000 per patient (unpublished data). Such an increase makes the large-scale application of these procedures not sustainable.

Paradoxically, the current NHS reimbursements do not enhance either the research and development applied by high-volume centers or the quality of the surgery provided. However, a long-term strategy should include also a reward for the quality of surgical outcomes, as defined by the value-based healthcare perspective [2]. Following this perspective, value is defined as the health outcomes achieved in relation to the cost of delivering these outcomes [3]. High-quality centers performing high-volume surgery should be recognized as centers of excellence and should receive adequate quality reimbursement.

17.3 The Issue of Data Sourcing

Another important issue concerns data sourcing. In general, any new initiative—especially within the scope of the NHS—should be the result of a process of data-driven decision-making. To date, the data supporting a positive relation between hospital volume and surgical outcome are derived from retrospective studies and central government databases, which use administrative codes for procedures that do not detail either the complexity of the operation or the complexity (i.e., the multimorbidity) of the patient undergoing the operation. Thus, any conclusion about quality outcome measures should be taken with caution. Perhaps, the new Observatory on Oncological Networks, which was established in 2019, will help in decoding the appropriate indicators to be used in such quality analyses (see Chap. 3).

17.4 The Importance of Centralization

The NHS operates, by definition, in a context of limited resources especially when central governments reduce the amount of resources allocated to the health services. In these conditions, rationalization of the organization of these services based on the volume of care may release resources to improve the effectiveness of interventions. The identification and certification of services and providers with high volume and quality of care can help to reduce differences in the access to high-quality procedures. However, whether the centralization of complex surgical procedures makes full sense being potentially associated with higher quality of care, as sometimes reported in the literature, precise criteria on what to centralize, where to centralize, and who should be entitled to perform complex procedures are still missing. Moreover, as previously reported, the hospital volume acts as a proxy measure for technical and nontechnical quality items that require being uncovered in specific elements [4–8]. Besides, there is a need for an accurate evaluation of the available scientific evidence in order to identify these standards, including the volume of care above or below which public and private hospitals may be accredited (or not) to provide specific health care interventions.

Since 2009, the National Outcomes Program (PNE, Piano Nazionale Esiti) has evaluated the outcomes of Italian hospitals [9]. As expected, the analysis of these data showed significant improvements in outcome measures in high-volume centers for the majority of the interventions recorded. In some cases, the improvement in outcomes remained gradual or constant with the increasing volume of care; in other cases, the analysis allowed the identification of threshold values beyond which the outcome does not improve further [9]. However, knowledge of the relationship between the effectiveness and costs of treatments and knowledge of the geographical distribution and accessibility to health care services are necessary for defining the minimum volumes of care, under which specific health procedures should be warranted. Yet, the "spending review" calls for the definition of "qualitative, structural, technological and quantitative standards of hospital care".

17.5 Volume Ranges in Oncological Surgery

Although there are currently no established hospital or surgeon volume thresholds linked to precise outcome levels, some volume ranges in oncological surgery might be extrapolated from the 2018 Italian National Outcomes Program. By way of example, we list here some data for selected malignancies, for the year 2017. It should be noted that the data should be read with caution: the details of the surgical procedures, the training history of the surgical team, the complexity of the tumor presentations, the multimorbidity of the patients, the appropriateness of the indication, and many other important features were not recorded and therefore cannot be extrapolated.

17.5.1 Gastric Cancer

In 2017, a total of 6239 surgical procedures for gastric cancer were performed: more than three procedures were performed in 358 surgical units, of which 81 (23%) had an activity volume of more than 20 procedures per year. The 30-day mortality rate was less than 10% when the hospital volume was more than 20–30 surgical procedures per year [9].

17.5.2 Pancreas Cancer

In pancreatic surgery, there is a consolidated association between volume and 30-day mortality: 30-day mortality after surgery significantly decreases when at least 50 surgical procedures per year are performed, and it continues to decrease for volumes higher than 50 procedures [3]. In 2017 in Italy, 2690 surgical procedures were performed for pancreatic cancer. However, only four Regions had at least one hospital with volumes higher than 50 procedures per year [9].

17.5.3 Colorectal Cancer

In 2017 in Italy, there were 26,784 patients with colorectal cancer. The 30-day mortality rate declines significantly as volumes rise up to 50–70 procedures per year; when the rise in volume exceeds this level, mortality continues to fall but at a slower rate [9]. Interestingly, the laparoscopic approach was adopted in 10,747 (40.1%) of cases. However, only 58 surgical units (11.7%) out of a total of 494 performed more than 50 laparoscopic procedures per year.

In 2017 in Italy, rectal cancer affected 6679 patients. Of these, 3118 were treated by laparoscopy (46.6%), but only 35 surgical units (9.75%) out of a total of 359 performed more than 20 laparoscopic procedures.

Of note, these rates of laparoscopic approach for colorectal cancer patients are increasing in comparison with previous records. However, they are still lower than in other European countries such as the United Kingdom, where a national training program has resulted in up to 60% of colorectal procedures being performed laparoscopically [10].

17.6 The Role of Italian Scientific Societies

In Italy, the two major Scientific Societies of General Surgery, ACOI (Associazione Chirurghi Ospedalieri Italiani) and SIC (Società Italiana di Chirurgia), have already developed dedicated programs to promote quality in surgical care throughout the country. Indeed, one of the strongholds of these Societies is the education and training of the member surgeons—especially young surgeons—with particular reference to the diffusion of a safety and quality culture, of new technologies, and of minimally invasive techniques. Besides, for many years these Societies have been working to define the competence of national centers of excellence, the training capacity of surgeons, and the clinical, surgical and scientific skills that should be set as minimum standard requirements.

17.7   Accreditation of Surgical Centers or Accreditation of Surgeons?

There is much discussion on the accreditation of surgical centers, which is no doubt a very important process in enhancing quality and safety. However, this process should be entrusted more to the regional or even central government bodies rather than to the Scientific Societies. Conversely, little has been said on the accreditation of the surgeons, although one strategy to improve quality, optimize human and technical resources, and eventually save public funds might be shifting attention from accreditation of the center to accreditation of the surgeon. This may prevent the paradox of having a given hospital or a given surgical department accredited for performing certain complex surgical procedures without having accredited expert surgeons: first the surgeons, then the department/hospital. In an age characterized by a tendency to level out knowledge, accrediting surgeons rather than hospital centers would mean giving professionals due recognition for their performance. Because surgery is still a craft, accreditation should concern first the craftsmen (surgeons) and then the workshops (hospitals). In this sense, shifting the current paradigm could lead to think more in terms of high-quality centers than high-volume centers. Similarly to the American Board of Surgery, which is an independent non-profit organization founded for the purpose of certifying surgeons who have met a defined standard of education, training and knowledge, the Italian Scientific Societies might work to define the minimum standard of care in major surgery on an individual basis with the aim of analyzing the applicant's training and surgical experience as well as his/her professionalism and ethics. After successful completion of these assessments, the surgeon might become certified in a specific field of major surgery. This certification might serve as a prerequisite of good practice which, combined with specific minimum requirements for the hospital as a single institution or as a network of institutions, might be a guarantee of high-quality care.

Moreover, the dualism between high volume and high quality has important limitations in Italy. Hitherto, there are 21 Regional Health Systems that differ in volumes and outcomes. These differences are determined by:

- high- and low-volume centers are not equally distributed across along the country;
- outdated and insufficient institutions, especially in the southern areas;
- difficult access to high-volume centers, which in general have longer waiting lists for diagnostic and therapeutic procedures;
- low penetrance of new techniques and technologies such as minimally invasive surgical procedures;
- inadequate surgical mentoring and training;
- failing recruiting strategies and policies by regional or central government agencies.

17.8 Call for Action

The centralization process as well as the accreditation of surgeons and departments requires close collaboration among governmental institutions, regional health systems and scientific societies/associations. The following main actions should be taken in consideration:

- definition of centers of excellence equally distributed across the country;
- revision at national and regional levels of the reimbursement system with the aim of favoring high-quality and high-volume centers;
- regional multidisciplinary pathways;
- continuous and advanced training, especially for new generations of surgeons;
- centralization of high-risk procedures;
- rigorous and modern surgical training with innovative methods and technologies;
- definition of accreditation criteria for surgeons and hospitals;
- monitoring of surgical performance;
- investments in high-quality centers, which are the centers of excellence.
- progressive acquisition and analyses of data in hospitals.

17.9 Conclusions

In conclusion, we believe that it is time for surgeons, clinicians and other health professionals to take these issues into their own hands so as to be the protagonists of change and not mere spectators. Every effort should be made to prevent the risk of the Italian National Health Service introducing new rules based on outcome-volume relationship not really data-driven, or anyway not adaptable to Italy. The current paradox of the reimbursement system should be taken as a general warning to avoid passing an outcome-volume paradox on to the next generations of surgeons and of patients.

References

1. Minami CA, Sheils CR, Bilimoria KY, et al. Process improvement in surgery. Curr Probl Surg. 2016;53(2):62–96.
2. Haas DA, Kaplan RS. Variation in the cost of care for primary total knee arthroplasties. Arthroplast Today. 2016;3(1):33–7.
3. Porter ME, Teisberg EO. Redefining health care: creating value-based competition on results. Boston, MA: Harvard Business School Press; 2006.
4. Mesman R, Faber MJ, Westert GP, Berden HJJM. Dutch surgeons' views on the volume-outcome mechanism in surgery: a qualitative interview study. Int J Qual Health Care. 2017;29(6):797–802.
5. Vonlanthen R, Lodge P, Barkun JS, et al. Toward a consensus on centralization in surgery. Ann Surg. 2018;268(5):712–24.

6. Morche J, Mathes T, Pieper D. Relationship between surgeon volume and outcomes: a systematic review of systematic reviews. Syst Rev. 2016;5(1):204. https://doi.org/10.1186/s13643-016-0376-4.
7. Gani F, Kim Y, Weiss MJ, et al. Effect of surgeon and anesthesiologist volume on surgical outcomes. J Surg Res. 2016;200(2):427–34.
8. Ravaioli M, Pinna AD, Francioni G, et al. A partnership model between high- and low-volume hospitals to improve results in hepatobiliary pancreatic surgery. Ann Surg. 2014;260(5):871–5.
9. Ministero della Salute—AGENAS. Piano Nazionale Esiti. https://pne.agenas.it.
10. Association of laparoscopic surgeons of Great Britain and Ireland. https://www.alsgbi.org.